BEHAVIORAL ACTIVATION WITH ADOLESCENTS

Also Available

Behavioral Activation for Depression:
A Clinician's Guide
*Christopher R. Martell, Sona Dimidjian,
and Ruth Herman-Dunn*

Behavioral Activation with Adolescents

A CLINICIAN'S GUIDE

Elizabeth McCauley
Kelly A. Schloredt
Gretchen R. Gudmundsen
Christopher R. Martell
Sona Dimidjian

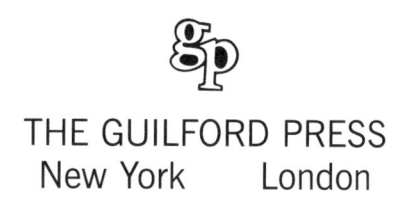

THE GUILFORD PRESS
New York   London

Copyright © 2016 The Guilford Press
A Division of Guilford Publications, Inc.
370 Seventh Avenue, Suite 1200, New York, NY 10001
www.guilford.com

All rights reserved

Except as indicated, no part of this book may be reproduced, translated, stored in a retrieval system, or transmitted, in any form or by any means, electronic, mechanical, photocopying, microfilming, recording, or otherwise, without written permission from the publisher.

Printed in the United States of America

This book is printed on acid-free paper.

Last digit is print number: 9   8   7   6   5   4   3   2   1

LIMITED DUPLICATION LICENSE

These materials are intended for use only by qualified mental health professionals.

The publisher grants to individual purchasers of this book nonassignable permission to reproduce all materials for which permission is specifically granted in a footnote. This license is limited to you, the individual purchaser, for personal use or use with individual clients. This license does not grant the right to reproduce these materials for resale, redistribution, electronic display, or any other purposes (including but not limited to books, pamphlets, articles, video- or audiotapes, blogs, file-sharing sites, Internet or intranet sites, and handouts or slides for lectures, workshops, webinars, or therapy groups, whether or not a fee is charged). Permission to reproduce these materials for these and any other purposes must be obtained in writing from the Permissions Department of Guilford Publications.

The authors have checked with sources believed to be reliable in their efforts to provide information that is complete and generally in accord with the standards of practice that are accepted at the time of publication. However, in view of the possibility of human error or changes in behavioral, mental health, or medical sciences, neither the authors, nor the editors and publisher, nor any other party who has been involved in the preparation or publication of this work warrants that the information contained herein is in every respect accurate or complete, and they are not responsible for any errors or omissions or the results obtained from the use of such information. Readers are encouraged to confirm the information contained in this book with other sources.

Library of Congress Cataloging-in-Publication Data

McCauley, Elizabeth, author.
  Behavioral activation with adolescents : a clinician's guide / by Elizabeth McCauley, Kelly A. Schloredt, Gretchen R. Gudmundsen, Christopher R. Martell, and Sona Dimidjian.
     pages cm
  Includes bibliographical references and index.
  ISBN 978-1-4625-2398-6 (pbk. : alk. paper)
   1. Depression in adolescence—Treatment.   2. Behavior therapy for teenagers.   I. Title.
RJ506.D4M3195 2016
616.85′2700835—dc23

2015030818

About the Authors

Elizabeth McCauley, PhD, ABPP, is Professor in the Department of Psychiatry and Behavioral Sciences at the University of Washington, with adjunct appointments in Psychology and Pediatrics, and Director of the Mood and Anxiety Program at Seattle Children's Hospital. Her clinical and research work focuses on the development and treatment of depression and suicidality in young people. Dr. McCauley has helped to lead two longitudinal studies tracking factors contributing to the onset and persistence of depression; has developed and tested a number of prevention and intervention strategies to treat or reduce the risk of depression and suicidality; and has led a project funded by the National Institute of Mental Health (NIMH) to test the efficacy of behavioral activation (BA) as a treatment for adolescent depression. She is a past president of the Society for Child and Adolescent Psychology and is board certified in clinical child and adolescent psychology through the American Board of Professional Psychology. Dr. McCauley has been actively involved in training through the University of Washington School of Medicine Psychology Internship Training Program and the Department of Psychology at the University of Washington.

Kelly A. Schloredt, PhD, ABPP, is Attending Clinical Psychologist in Child Psychiatry and Behavioral Medicine and Clinical Director of the Psychiatry and Behavioral Medicine Unit at Seattle Children's Hospital, as well as Clinical Professor of Psychiatry in the Department of Psychiatry and Behavioral Sciences at the University of Washington. She is board certified in clinical child and adolescent psychology through the American Board of Professional Psychology and is actively engaged in a range of professional activities, including management and administration, teaching, patient care, and supervision and training. Dr. Schloredt was a research therapist on the Adolescent BA Program study (led by Elizabeth McCauley) and has worked on a number of NIMH-funded research projects related to depression in youth.

Gretchen R. Gudmundsen, PhD, is Assistant Professor in the Department of Psychiatry and Behavioral Sciences at the University of Washington and Attending Clinical Psychologist in Child Psychiatry and Behavioral Medicine at Seattle Children's Hospital. She has published numerous articles on the treatment of depression and on the role of stress and coping in depressive disorders. Dr. Gudmundsen provides direct outpatient care in addition to providing supervision and training. A recipient of a Klingenstein Third Generation Foundation Fellowship for Child and Adolescent Depression, she has been a research therapist on several NIMH-funded research projects on the treatment of adolescent mood disorders.

Christopher R. Martell, PhD, ABPP, is Clinical Professor in the Department of Psychology at the University of Wisconsin–Milwaukee and the owner of Martell Behavioral Activation Research Consulting. He maintained an independent practice for 23 years, providing cognitive-behavioral therapy to clients with mood and anxiety disorders. Dr. Martell has conducted workshops and trainings on BA nationally and internationally and has consulted on research teams examining BA around the world. He is board certified in cognitive and behavioral psychology and in clinical psychology through the American Board of Professional Psychology. Dr. Martell is a recipient of several honors, including the Distinguished Psychologist Award from the Washington State Psychological Association, and is the coauthor of several books, including *Behavioral Activation for Depression: A Clinician's Guide*.

Sona Dimidjian, PhD, is Associate Professor in the Department of Psychology and Neuroscience at the University of Colorado Boulder. Her research addresses the treatment and prevention of depression, with a particular focus on the mental health of women during pregnancy and postpartum. Dr. Dimidjian is a leading expert on behavioral approaches to depression, as well as the clinical application of contemplative practices, such as mindfulness meditation. She has a long-standing interest in the dissemination of empirically supported treatments and evidence-based practice, both nationally and internationally. Dr. Dimidjian's teaching and clinical research have been recognized with numerous awards, including the Dorothy Martin Women's Faculty Award, the Outstanding Graduate Mentor Award from the University of Colorado Boulder, and the Susan A. Hickman Memorial Research Award from Postpartum Support International.

Acknowledgments

We would like to express our enthusiastic thanks to the people who made this book possible. First and foremost, many thanks to The Guilford Press team—Kitty Moore, Carolyn Graham, Louise Farkas, and their colleagues—who supported us with kindness, respect, and infinite patience. It has been an honor and privilege to work with all of you. We would also like to thank the Psychiatry and Behavioral Medicine Department and the Research Institute at Seattle Children's Hospital for supporting us in countless ways and providing an intellectually stimulating and nurturing environment for our treatment development efforts. Our work was supported by funding from the National Institute of Mental Health (R34MH076956), the University of Washington/Seattle Children's Hospital ITHS Pediatric Clinical Research Center and National Center for Research Resources (UL1RR025014), and the Seattle Children's Research Institute. Finally, and most important, we would like to thank the adolescents and parents who partnered with us in this collaborative endeavor—you guided our work each step of the way and made it meaningful. Simply stated, without the support and contributions of each of these key groups, the work represented in this book would not have been possible—so three cheers of thanks to all!

Elizabeth McCauley: I offer thanks to my coauthors. Together we transformed, albeit painstakingly, a vague notion that we could "do better" into a theoretically based, evidence-informed, and clinically useful set of intervention strategies. Perseverance does pay off, and thanks to all of you for hanging in there. I would also like to acknowledge my husband, Emory Hill, whose support and friendship nurtures and sustains me.

Kelly A. Schloredt: I would also like to acknowledge and offer thanks to my coauthors, particularly Elizabeth McCauley, for providing me with endless opportunities over the course of my career, for inviting me to be part of the behavioral activation (BA) team, and for leading us through this endeavor. Although the process has been long and challenging, it has been an intellectually stimulating, thought-provoking, enjoyable, and collaborative effort that I would not trade for anything. I cannot think of a better group of people with whom to have shared this journey. I would also like to acknowledge my mother, Sharon Schloredt Plihal, for her ongoing support and encouragement and my deceased father, Ben Schloredt, whose words upon my acceptance into graduate school—"I think writing a book someday would be a good idea"—I have never forgotten. I know this book would have made him extraordinarily proud!

Gretchen R. Gudmundsen: I wish to thank each of my coauthors for welcoming me to the BA team, first as a postdoctoral fellow and eventually as a faculty colleague. Their mentorship and expertise has shaped my development as a psychologist. Adolescent depression is challenging, and I am thrilled to share what we've learned with other therapists and the youth and families they serve. I am grateful for the support and patience of my husband, Jason Prantner. Over the course of working on this book, we welcomed to our family Max and Hattie (who got to spend a lot of extra time with Dad when Mom needed to write).

Christopher R. Martell: I would first like to acknowledge my coauthors of this manual. Our weekly conversations, supervision team meetings, and writing sessions were a highlight of my Friday afternoons, and occasional weekends, for many years. I know much more about treating children and adolescents now than when we began. As always, I also would like to acknowledge the brilliant work and generosity of the late Neil S. Jacobson for bringing me into his Treatments for Depression Study and allowing me to help develop contemporary BA. Finally, I am always grateful for the support and advice that Steven Hollon has provided through the years on all of our BA projects. Steve is the finest example of an inquisitive scientist, open to whatever story the data have to tell, and he is a cherished colleague and friend.

Sona Dimidjian: I express heartfelt thanks to my coauthors, an inspiring and dedicated group of collaborators with whom I have been delighted and honored to work. I also acknowledge the influence of my late mentor Neil S. Jacobson on my work and on the field. His unwavering commitment to the value of behavioral approaches to depression helped to set us all on a course that has touched the lives of many. And, like Christopher, I want to acknowledge Steven Hollon, my most generous adoptive mentor and friend, who has helped to ensure that our work on BA has continued with the highest integrity. Finally, I express my gratitude to my daughter, Serena, who continually reminds me of the joy that is available at all stages of life, including adolescence, and of the importance of doing this work.

Preface

Emotional and behavioral health problems are common in children and adolescents, affecting as many as one in five youth (Costello, Foley, & Angold, 2006). They represent the most costly health condition of childhood (Soni, 2009) and impede successful school engagement and social development. Thus, the need for effective mental health care for youth is pressing. Fortunately, the field of child and adolescent mental health has made tremendous progress over the last 10 to 15 years. Effective intervention approaches for treating many emotional and behavioral problems in youth have been developed, tested, and proven to be beneficial, and at least two effective interventions for adolescent depression, cognitive-behavioral therapy (CBT) and interpersonal psychotherapy for adolescents (IPT-A), have been identified. Many youth, however, do not receive such interventions, in part because the sheer number and complexity of approaches now available to therapists make implementation and dissemination of these evidence-based treatments challenging. To address this problem, Chorpita and Daleiden (2009) have begun to tease out the elements common to many interventions that may be most useful in helping to improve youth mental health. It is in the context of contributing to these ongoing efforts to both improve and simplify treatment of adolescent depression that we present our work on behavioral activation (BA). Our approach focuses on drawing on these common elements to outline straightforward intervention strategies that we believe clinicians can readily integrate into their practice and that are accessible to depressed youth.

Clinical need coupled with a bit of chance triggered our interest in adapting BA as a way of working with adolescents struggling with depression. Our team came to this work well steeped in CBT, having used this approach for years with children or adults. In our experience, introducing the cognitive triangle and working with clients to recognize and challenge automatic negative thoughts worked well for many adolescents, but not for all. More specifically, we found that such strategies were particularly difficult for our adolescent clients, who seemed to consider questions about their thinking as challenges to their beliefs about themselves—as if we, their therapists, were discounting their feelings, thoughts, and beliefs. Along these same lines, the CBT approach that starts with a focus on encouraging adolescents to be more engaged in pleasant events also made sense but did not work readily with many unmotivated adolescents, who did not seem to see the worth or "payoff" in trying something new or even talking with a friend. Furthermore, the important interpersonal and social communication component of IPT-A seemed missing from standard CBT protocols. As we struggled together to think about how to improve our skills, a number of other important and somewhat chance events coalesced around us.

One such event was the explosion of neuroscience research on adolescent brain development, which confirmed what we always suspected—adolescents do think and react differently from adults! These findings underscored the need to more directly address avoidance and reward responsivity. At the same time, two of us (Sona Dimidjian and Christopher R. Martell) were engaged in conducting a large study testing BA with depressed adults. When results from this work suggested that BA could hold up as a "stand-alone" treatment, we quickly recognized that it offered an approach that might just fit the needs of our adolescents. Specifically, BA offered a focused and in-depth consideration of what activities are associated with feeling positive or feeling down and what was getting in the way of more or complete engagement in activities that brought adolescents a sense of well-being and purpose. In addition, the BA model offered a nonthreatening and pragmatic stance that we felt would enhance engagement in treatment and motivate our clients to experiment with trying something new. Finally, BA impressed us as a straightforward approach that would be easy for the adolescent to embrace and the therapist to learn. Thus we joined forces as an integrated team of experts in child and adolescent depression and behavioral activation.

The Adolescent Behavioral Activation Program (A-BAP) was developed from this base. We present this approach as a way to complement other efforts to support adolescents dealing with depression, as well as other behavioral health concerns. This treatment manual outlines a session-by-session approach in order to give the therapist a clear overview and guidelines. Our approach was developed in an iterative manner. We began with a series of individual case trials; actively elicited feedback from our adolescent clients, parents, and fellow therapists; and incorporated their suggestions. Throughout this process, we made a number of revisions to the manual and ultimately conducted a small randomized clinical study (McCauley et al., 2015). The A-BAP approach proved effective in reducing depressive symptoms in the majority of adolescent participants, and initial coding indicated that therapists were able to deliver the intervention as outlined with adherence. The collection of research and clinical evidence regarding the efficacy of a BA approach is ongoing, with studies in progress in the United States and England, as well as clinical work using the BA approach with youth who have anxiety and other health concerns.

In this manual we also emphasize the ways that BA strategies can be integrated effectively with other treatment approaches. Adolescents struggling with depression are a varied group of individuals. For some, depression is triggered by significant interpersonal conflict, for others by a negative thinking bias, and for still others by having lost the motivation to engage in what were once rewarding activities. Over the next decade, we are confident that research will reveal differential pathways to depression among adolescents and help us to identify specific subtypes within the heterogeneous category of "adolescent depression." We predict, however, that BA strategies will be essential, in some form, in any effective therapeutic work with depressed adolescents. BA is well suited to youth with motivational deficits. For youth who may benefit from the addition of interpersonal or cognitive strategies, BA also may be a good "starting point" as a way to engage them in either CBT or IPT-A, two strategies proven effective for treating adolescent depression.

We have spent a significant amount of our clinical and research time over the past decade refining this approach and developing the manual. We hope that you will find the structure of this manual easy to use and the strategies outlined beneficial to your work with adolescents.

Contents

Chapter 1. Depression and Behavioral Activation with Adolescents — 1

Chapter 2. Assessment, Case Conceptualization, and Treatment Planning — 24

Chapter 3. How to Use the A-BAP Session Guides — 43

Chapter 4. Management of Treatment Challenges within the A-BAP Approach — 59

Chapter 5. Applications of Behavioral Activation with Other Clinical Samples/Situations — 75

A-BAP Treatment Sessions

MODULE 1. GETTING STARTED

Session 1. Introduction to the Adolescent Behavioral Activation Program (A-BAP) — 91

Session 2. Situation–Activity–Mood Cycle — 97

MODULE 2. GETTING ACTIVE

Session 3. Goal-Directed Behavior versus Mood-Directed Behavior — 107

Session 4. Introducing Consequences of Behavior — 114

MODULE 3. SKILL BUILDING

Session 5. Problem Solving — 123

Session 6. Goal Setting — 131

Session 7. Identifying Barriers — 138

Session 8. Overcoming Avoidance — 145

MODULE 4. PRACTICE

Session 9. Putting It All Together — 155

Sessions 10 and 11. Practicing Skills — 160

MODULE 5. MOVING FORWARD

Session 12. Relapse Prevention and Saying Good-Bye — 167

Reproducible Handouts — 173

References — 213

Index — 223

Purchasers of this book can download and print the handouts at *www.guilford.com/mccauley-forms* for personal use or use with individual clients (see copyright page for details).

CHAPTER 1

Depression and Behavioral Activation with Adolescents

The Adolescent Behavioral Activation Program (A-BAP) utilizes a behavioral activation (BA) approach to treating depressed adolescents. Designed for adolescents between the ages of 12 and 18, the program typically consists of 12–14 sessions, organized in five modules, and is typically delivered once a week. Although the program is structured, it is designed to be used flexibly following the principles of BA. This treatment manual includes detailed, session-by-session instructions for therapists, as well as handouts for the adolescent and the parent(s) in treatment. Parents are actively involved in the treatment and are oriented to the BA model, educated about depression, and taught strategies to improve communication with the adolescent and ways to support the adolescent's treatment goals. We fully acknowledge the diversity of families and living situations and use the word *parent* throughout to indicate an adult or adults who are actively involved in the life of the adolescent, and who have the legal right to participate in his or her treatment.

The A-BAP approach to treating depression was modified from behavioral activation treatment as developed for adult depression (Martell, Addis, & Jacobson, 2001). Chapters 1–5 of this volume cover background and implementation of the treatment program. In this chapter (Chapter 1), we provide an overview of our understanding of the impact of depression on adolescents, a review of current treatment findings, a description of the behavioral model of depression, and an overview of the A-BAP approach. In Chapter 2, we discuss assessment, case conceptualization, and treatment planning. Chapter 3 provides a hands-on, session-by-session guide to implementing the material in the A-BAP manual. Chapter 4 considers strategies for handling challenges that often arise in treatment, such as suicidal behaviors, and Chapter 5 explores how the A-BAP might be used effectively with other clinical problems or populations, such as youth coping with anxiety or chronic pain. The actual treatment protocol, including session-by-session outlines of the five modules, follows. The final section consists of handouts to support each session.

The Problem of Depression in Adolescence

Most therapists working with adolescents treat youth with depression or other psychiatric or medical disorders that are complicated by depression. Adolescent depression is widely recognized as a major public health problem (Lopez, Mathers, Ezzati, Jamison, & Murray, 2006). Population-based prevalence rates indicate that at any point in time, 0.4–8.3% of adolescents are struggling with depression, and cumulative prevalence rates suggest that 20% of youth have at least one episode of clinical depression by age 18 (Costello, Egger, & Angold, 2005; Hankin et al., 1998; Lewinsohn, Clarke, Seeley, & Rohde, 1994). Moreover, relapse and recurrence of depression are common. Following an episode of depression, approximately 50–70% of depressed youth experience a relapse within 2 to 5 years of diagnosis, and these youth are at increased risk for recurring depression in adulthood (Curry et al., 2011; Dunn & Goodyer, 2006; Goodyer, Herbert, Tamplin, & Altham, 2000; Lewinsohn, Rohde, Seeley, Klein, & Gotlib, 2000). It is further estimated that 65% of youth experience transient or less severe depressive symptoms during their adolescent years (Lewinsohn, Hops, Roberts, Seeley, & Andrews, 1993); however, studies suggest that even subclinical symptoms of depression are associated with adverse consequences (Fergusson, Horwood, Ridder, & Beautrais, 2005; Lewinsohn, Solomon, Seeley, & Zeiss, 2000). Depression in adolescence represents a risk for substance use and suicide, and more generally compromises psychosocial development and interferes with academic achievement, as well as peer and family relationships (Keenan-Miller, Hammen, & Brennan, 2007). Moreover, long-term sequelae of adolescent depression include a host of broader functional deficits, such as poor global and adaptive functioning, and academic and occupational impairment (Copeland, Shanahan, Costello, & Angold, 2009; Fergusson & Woodward, 2002; Glied & Pine, 2002; Lewinsohn, Rohde, Seeley, Klein, & Gotlib, 2003). These far-reaching consequences underscore the importance of identifying effective prevention and intervention approaches.

Developmental factors may contribute to the increased risk for depression in adolescents. Adolescence is a time of significant neurocognitive development, reorganization, and structural change (e.g., Giedd et al., 1999; Gould & Tanapat, 1999; Hare et al., 2008; Luna, Padmanabhan, & O'Hearn, 2010; Somerville, Jones, & Casey, 2010). Adolescents experience heightened emotionality, perhaps secondary to the hormonal changes of puberty, which can hamper their ability to mobilize executive functioning skills, such as impulse and emotion control, memory, self-monitoring, and planning abilities. They demonstrate limited abilities to process complex tasks due to an immature working memory and an inability to inhibit impulsive responses (response inhibition) (Crone, Wendelken, Donohue, van Leijenhorst, & Bunge, 2006; Steinberg et al., 2006; Velanova, Wheeler, & Luna, 2008). The structural brain changes that lay the foundation for more sophisticated skills, such as response inhibition, problem solving, and long-term planning, do not fully develop until late adolescence or early adulthood (Casey, Duhoux,

& Cohen, 2010; Giedd, 2004). The gap between the increase in emotional or affective response during early adolescence and the development of neuroregulatory mechanisms (Davey, Yücel, & Allen, 2008) contributes to problems with affect regulation. This leaves many adolescents vulnerable to biased interpretations of experiences, self-criticism, low inhibitory control, and emotion-focused coping (Giedd et al., 1999; Luna et al., 2010)—all variables that are correlated with depression. Moreover, the brain reactivity of depressed adolescents may differ in important ways from the brain reactivity of depressed adults. Although depressed adults demonstrate increased and sustained physiological reactivity to emotional information, ==depressed and anxious adolescents demonstrate decreased reactivity, suggesting a shutting down or avoidance of emotional stimuli== (Silk et al., 2007). Additional evidence suggests that disruption of reward processing may be part of the physiological changes that contribute to depression regardless of age, and that vulnerability to reward dysregulation may be greater during adolescence because neural reward systems are still developing (Davey et al., 2008; Forbes, 2009).

Awareness of the neurocognitive changes affecting the adolescent brain may inform the development and selection of optimally effective intervention strategies. Research findings suggest that treatment for adolescent depression may need to target the adolescent's ability to (1) ==experience and respond to reward==, and (2) ==overcome avoidance==—both targets that are key components of behavioral activation (Forbes, 2009).

Current Approaches to Treating Adolescent Depression

Most research on the treatment of adolescent depression has focused on the efficacy of cognitive-behavioral therapy (CBT), interpersonal therapy (IPT), and pharmacotherapies, alone or in combination. Both CBT and IPT utilize a short-term therapy approach, with a focus on the "here and now" rather than the past; in both, the therapist plays an active role in providing education about depression and engaging adolescents in structured steps and skill building to reduce their depressive symptoms. Although the findings for both approaches have been promising, treatment challenges persist.

CBT treatments for adolescent depression, modified from adult CBT treatment programs, have been utilized for many years (Clarke, DeBar, Ludman, Asarnow, & Jaycox, 2002; Lewinsohn, Clarke, Hops, & Andrews, 1990). They include behavioral interventions such as scheduling pleasant activities, problem solving, and relaxation, and they focus centrally on cognitive elements, such as the positive restructuring of negative thoughts (i.e., cognitive restructuring) and examining and challenging underlying beliefs. Although early CBT findings in youth were very positive, recent studies suggest a more muted and delayed response pattern. The Treatment of Adolescents with Depression Study (TADS), for example, found that at immediate posttreatment (12 weeks), adolescents randomized to CBT did not differ from those in the pill-placebo control group and had a significantly lower response rate than adolescents randomized to fluoxetine alone or CBT and fluoxetine combined (TADS Team, 2004). At the 36-week follow-up evaluation, however, the effects of CBT alone and fluoxetine alone converged with those of combined treatment, indicating significant improvement in symptoms for approximately

80% of the participants (TADS Team, 2007). This positive response rate close to a year posttreatment may reflect, in part, the natural course of depression given evidence that depressive episodes remit in most adolescents (60–90%) within 1 year (Thapar, Collishaw, Pine, & Thapar, 2012). As noted earlier, however, recurrence rates remain high, suggesting limits to persistent treatment efficacy.

IPT modified for adolescents (IPT-A) also has demonstrated promising efficacy (Mufson, Weissman, Moreau, & Garfinkel, 1999; Rosselló, & Bernal, 1999) at posttreatment and at 16-week follow-up, as well as in initial effectiveness testing in school-based health clinics (Mufson et al., 2004; Young, Mufson, & Davies, 2006; Mufson, Dorta, Moreau, & Weissman, 2011). IPT conceptualizes depression as a medical illness in an effort to reduce the sense of self-blame that often accompanies it and focuses on the interaction among mood, life events, and interpersonal relationships as key maintenance factors of depressive symptoms. IPT, therefore, focuses on enhancing communication skills using strategies such as encouragement of affect, role playing, and communication analyses to address challenges of role transitions and interpersonal problems as a way to improve the adolescent's relationships and thereby reduce depressive symptoms. This approach has been particularly effective for youth with social dysfunction and parent–child conflict (Gunlicks-Stoessel, Mufson, Jekal, & Turner, 2010; Mufson et al., 1999, 2004). Comprehensive evaluation of IPT-A, however, has been hindered by small sample sizes, the absence of data on long-term outcome and relapse rates, and lack of comparison, singly or in combination, to antidepressant medication (Mufson, 2010).

Parent involvement in the treatment of adolescent depression varies widely. While both CBT and IPT-A employ an individual therapy approach, CBT interventions frequently involve coaching parents to reinforce therapeutic interventions or may include directly teaching parents strategies for parenting, conflict resolution, or communication. IPT-A includes parent psychoeducation in all phases of care and works actively with parents and adolescents together on communication and problem solving when indicated to help improve the adolescent's mood (Mufson et al., 2004). A renewed interest in testing interventions that include a significant family or parent component has emerged over the last decade. Prior findings on the efficacy of including a parental component to treatment for depression have been mixed, but in a recent meta-analysis of treatment across diagnoses, inclusion of a parent–child combined approach yielded a moderate benefit over and above that achieved by individual child treatments (Dowell & Ogles, 2010). Attachment-based family therapy (ABFT; Diamond & Josephson, 2005; Diamond et al., 2010; Israel & Diamond, 2013), based on interpersonal theory, posits that rebuilding interpersonal relationships within families can lead to reductions in depression and suicidality in adolescents. Results from a series of small studies of ABFT suggest clinically significant reductions in depressive symptoms and self-reported suicidal ideation. ABFT is seen as a "promising" intervention approach (David-Ferdon & Kaslow, 2008), and its success underscores the need to revisit parental involvement in treatment of adolescent depression.

Finally, even though pharmacotherapy alone has been shown to benefit approximately 60% of youth and close to 70% of youth when combined with CBT, it has been associated with controversy. Introduction of a new class of antidepressants, the selective serotonin reuptake inhibitors (SSRIs), in the 1990s, marked a dramatic increase in the prescription of antidepressants to children and adolescents. This rise in the use of SSRIs has presumably occurred because these medications are considered "safe"; they do not have high lethality with overdose or the cardiac side effects found with early antidepressant medication. In 2004, however, the U.S. Food and Drug Administration (FDA) issued a "black box" warning regarding the use of antidepressants with youth due to mood-related side effects, specifically, increases in suicidal thoughts and behaviors (Moreland, Bonin, Brent, & Solomon, 2014). This warning triggered an ongoing debate about the use of antidepressant medications with young people. The data on medication-triggered suicidality has been controversial (Brent & Birmaher, 2004; Mann et al., 2006; Nemeroff et al., 2007), and many stress the idea that emergent suicidality is simply a core risk in all treatment of adolescent depression—psychopharmacology or psychotherapy (Bridge, Barbe, Birmaher, Kolko, & Brent, 2005). Furthermore, a recent meta-analysis of 17 studies of the use of antidepressants in children and adolescents found significant increases in emotional arousal and behavior activation in youth taking antidepressants compared to placebo controls (Offidani, Fava, Tomba, & Baldessarini, 2013). With that said, however, care guidelines are clear about the need to educate adolescents and parents regarding the risk of escalating thoughts of suicide, regularly monitoring suicidality, and engaging in active outreach as indicated (Simon, 2006).

Following the FDA warning, there has been a 25–58% drop in antidepressant prescriptions (Libby et al., 2007; Libby, Orton, & Valuck, 2009). The use of pharmacological interventions for depressed youth is also influenced by many adolescents' negative attitudes about medication use (Williams, Hollis, & Benoit, 1998); many adolescents for whom medications are prescribed fail to receive an adequate treatment trial because they do not take medication as prescribed or they discontinue its use prematurely (Richardson, DiGiuseppe, Christakis, McCauley, & Katon, 2004; Richardson & Katzenellenbogen, 2005). The decline in medication use has in turn led to concern about inadequate treatment of depression and subsequent increases in suicide rates, with reports of a 14% increase in youth suicide in the United States between 2003 and 2004—the largest year-to-year increase in youth suicide rates since 1979 (Gibbons et al., 2007; Simon, 2006). Taken together, these findings suggest that viable alternatives or adjuncts to medication approaches are warranted.

Of great concern is the fact that a significant subset of youth does not respond to any type of treatment, even combined therapy. This was exemplified in the TADS, in which approximately 50% of youth had significant residual symptoms following the initial 12-week treatment, and overall remission (as opposed to response) rates were only 60% by the 36-week follow-up evaluation (Kennard et al., 2006, 2009). Furthermore, it is clear that some subgroups of adolescents are at particularly high risk for poor response to treatment, such as those exposed to early life adversity (Lewis et al., 2010; Nanni, Uher, & Danese, 2012). Even considering adolescents generally, it is clear that more robust interventions are needed. In a recently completed meta-analysis, Weisz and colleagues (2013) compared evidence-based therapies for a variety of child/adolescent mental health problems, including depression, with treatment as usual (TAU). Although evidence-based therapies, including CBT and IPT, were associated with better outcomes when compared to TAU, the effect size across studies was modest and less robust among youth who actually met diagnostic criteria for a disorder.

It is possible that response to current treatments is limited by a reliance on strategies that are a developmental mismatch for some adolescents. The mechanism of action in CBT is thought to be the remediation of biased cognitive processing through cognitive restructuring. Biased cognitive processing refers to the negative thinking or interpretation of events that commonly comes with feeling depressed. Cognitive restructuring first involves pointing out that what and/or how we think affects how we feel, and in turn, what we do (cognitive triangle), and second, involves working with the adolescent to come up with alternative thoughts that give rise to more neutral or positive feelings (DeRubeis, Siegle, & Hollon, 2008; Siegle, Steinhauer, Friedman, Thompson, & Thase, 2011). For IPT-A, the mechanism of change is thought to be improved social skills and relationships. Both approaches rely on the adolescent effectively learning and implementing sophisticated cognitive and interpersonal skills. Mastery of these skills, however, may be difficult for a substantial subset of adolescents who have not yet developed the cognitive maturity or competence needed for cognitive restructuring, interpersonal problem solving, including the ability to take another person's perspective, and response inhibition, particularly in the face of increased emotional arousal.

One response to concerns about the possible mismatch between complex strategies and the capacities of adolescents has been the development of more modularized approaches to treatment. These approaches, such as the Practice Wise Managing and Adapting Practice system (MAP; Chorpita & Daleiden, 2009), involve the systematic matching of youth mental health problems and demographic characteristics to associated treatment elements (or modules) that have been identified in the scientific literature as components of empirically supported interventions for particular demographic and diagnostic groups. MAP is based on the distillation and matching model, which states that evidence-based psychosocial interventions can be distilled into sets of content elements, then matched to client problems and individual characteristics (Chorpita, Daleiden, & Weisz, 2005). MAP was developed to simplify the process by which mental health therapists select and implement a treatment plan within busy community-based settings. This approach enables a therapist to deliver treatment elements in each session that are most likely to promote change, thereby increasing the chance that even a small treatment dose might be effective. Weisz and colleagues (2012) have reported that the modularized approach is associated with greater symptom reduction than usual care or standard manualized treatments (CBT for depression and anxiety, behavioral parent training for externalizing problems) in a randomized trial with 174 children between ages 7 and 13. The efficacy of the modular approach underscores the importance of identifying treatment elements that can facilitate treatments tailored to an individual's specific needs and circumstances. It is possible that treatment responses of depressed adolescents might also be improved by focusing on strategies that target the specific functional deficits associated with adolescent development described earlier in this chapter (Forbes, 2009; Forbes et al., 2009). These considerations motivated us to consider testing the value of BA components in the treatment of adolescents.

The BA Model of Depression

BA is based on a behavioral model of depression (Ferster, 1973; see Figure 1.1), which emphasizes the importance of considering positive reinforcement and punishment in the environment, and the function that depressive behaviors serve in an individual's life. The approach is idiographic, considering the specific context in each case to determine possible factors contributing to the depressive behaviors, those that serve to maintain it, and the behaviors/events required to treat it. Two interrelated concepts are central to the theory of change in BA. First is the idea that an individual needs to have the opportunity to experience positive reinforcement for adaptive behavior from his or her environment, and second is the idea that avoidance is a common barrier to engaging in adaptive behavior. Pleasant events scheduling is frequently included in CBT approaches as a strategy to boost mood by encouraging withdrawn individuals to reengage in social and physical activities; this component of CBT has more recently been referred to as *behavioral activation*. Within the CBT model, however, pleasant events scheduling or BA typically follows a nomothetic approach, identifying activities that "should" be pleasant to most people. As noted earlier, however, BA takes a more idiographic approach to identifying the specific events that may both trigger and maintain depression for each individual, countering this cycle by building in specific, rewarding responses/activities to these triggers, with attention to overcoming avoidance that may maintain a negative response cycle. Avoidance behavior often offers short-term symptom relief but is maintained via negative reinforcement (i.e., the strengthening of behavior via removal of a noxious stimulus), therefore serving to maintain depression in the long run. Although avoidance was recognized as central to depression, as well as anxiety disorders, in the early 1970s (Ferster, 1973), treatments for depression, such as CBT and IPT, have not identified avoidance behaviors as primary treatment targets. In this way, the emphasis on avoidance behaviors in the current BA model is unique. BA focuses on providing an in-depth focus on understanding how events in a person's life may both trigger and maintain depression, and the role of avoidance in maintaining this negative response cycle.

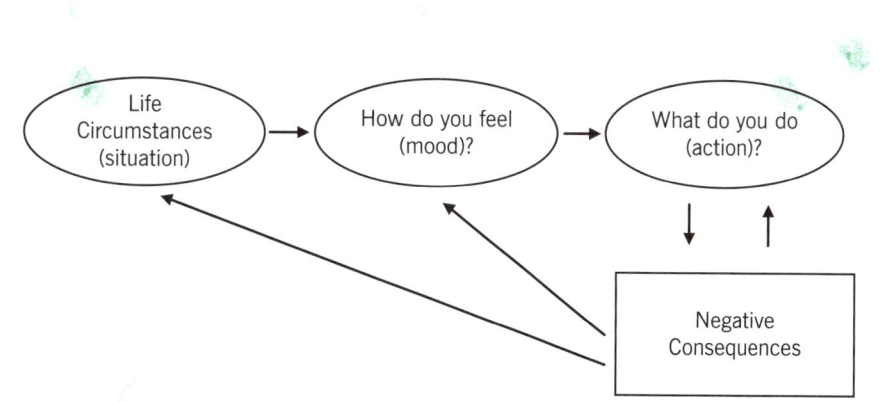

FIGURE 1.1. The BA model of depression.

BA for Adult Depression

In their work on adult depression treatment, Jacobson and colleagues (1996) conducted a component analysis of Beck's cognitive therapy (CT) for depression (Beck, Rush, Shaw, & Emery, 1979). They explored whether the simpler BA component of CT would work as well as the full CT approach that included both behavioral and cognitive interventions. To the surprise of many, the BA component alone worked as well as the full CT approach, and a larger trial was initiated, with BA articulated as a treatment in its own right (Jacobson, Martell, & Dimidjian, 2001; Martell et al., 2001). In this trial, BA was compared with CT, antidepressant medication, and a pill-placebo condition. Results indicated that among more severely depressed adults, BA worked as well as antidepressant medication and had some advantage over CT (Dimidjian et al., 2006). BA for adults is an idiographic approach wherein the therapist works under the umbrella of a behavioral case conceptualization and conducts an analysis of each client's life situation, goals, and the function of his or her daily activities, with a particular emphasis on identifying behaviors that function as avoidance and maintain depressive symptoms. The standard session structure of CBT—namely, identifying treatment goals, collaboratively setting an agenda for each session, and assigning and reviewing homework—is followed, but the treatment strategies utilized with individual clients in BA vary based on the functional analysis and individual client needs.

Why BA for Adolescents?

BA may also represent a promising approach for depressed adolescents. BA targets engagement with possible reinforcers within the adolescent's environment and may be one strategy to enhance outcomes. BA also is consistent with the understanding of adolescent development emerging from recent findings in cognitive and affective neuroscience. The focus on activation is highly compatible with the developmental needs and abilities of adolescents. Unlike existing therapies that call on sophisticated and higher-order cognitive concepts, BA is an idiographic, behavioral approach that uniquely centers on (1) activation to increase a youth's probability of exposure to naturally rewarding experiences, (2) identification and reduction of barriers to activation, and (3) recognition of avoidance patterns coupled with generation of alternative coping strategies that potentiate the experience of reward for the individual adolescent.

Moreover, excitement about BA has been driven by the belief that since it relies on a few basic treatment strategies, it is relatively easy to learn and administer effectively. The emerging field of implementation science suggests that barriers to utilizing evidence-based treatments in real-world settings include the therapist's lack of knowledge and skills in applying available interventions (Garland et al., 2010; Palinkas et al., 2008). The ease of learning and using new treatment approaches is enhanced with a simplified treatment design (Aarons & Chaffin, 2013; Rotheram-Borus, Swendeman, & Chorpita, 2012). There is concern that CBT is difficult to disseminate because of the finding that outcomes differ based on treatment location, even in highly controlled research trials

(DeRubeis et al., 2005), and others have noted that CBT can be difficult to teach and administer with fidelity (Kerfoot, Harrington, Harrington, Rogers, & Verduyn, 2004; Weisz, Jensen, & McLeod, 2005). Efforts to deliver CBT in TADS (TADS Team, 2004, 2007), the largest study to date on the treatment of adolescent depression, yielded disappointing results, with CBT not consistently outperforming pharmacological intervention, even with resource-intensive training and supervision (TADS Team, 2003). Subsequent efforts to understand the disappointing performance of CBT in TADS have emphasized the potential problems with using multiple intervention strategies, which precluded sufficient practice and mastery of core skills (Hollon, Garber, & Shelton, 2005). In contrast, BA's focus on only a few core behavioral strategies allows time for repeated skills application and practice tailored to the individualized needs of each adolescent. BA does not introduce too many strategies and does not depend on mastery of complex cognitive components. Thus, it is possible that it may be effectively used by a wide range of providers with varying education and experience levels and practiced in diverse settings, including community mental health centers, schools, and primary care settings in which caseloads are high, resources are limited, and time is at a premium. BA's potential for rapid uptake into clinical practice also supports its relevance for therapists working with depressed adolescents.

Does BA for Adolescent Depression Work?

Initial studies with adolescents using BA adapted to target avoidant behaviors at home, at school, and with peers, have been promising (Chu, Colognori, Weissman, & Bannon, 2009; Jacob, Keeley, Ritschel, & Craighead, 2013; Ritschel, Ramirez, Jones, & Craighead, 2011). Ritschel and colleagues (Jacob et al., 2013; Ritschel et al., 2011) tested the efficacy of the BA approach in two open trials with a small but ethnically diverse group of adolescents and documented significant improvement in depressive symptoms, such that the majority of participants no longer met criteria for depression at the end of their course of treatment (e.g., up to 17 sessions). Likewise, Chu and his team (2009) reported support for the feasibility and efficacy of using a group-based BA approach within the school setting for young adolescents struggling with anxiety and/or depression. Our own research group has shown that our A-BAP approach, based on the adult BA approach, can be delivered successfully, with efficacy, to depressed adolescents. In our study, the A-BAP was evaluated in comparison to a very robust TAU condition in which skilled therapists provided either CBT- or IPT-based care. While we anticipated that there would be a positive response in the TAU condition, we wanted to determine whether the A-BAP would result in an equally positive treatment response. Youth in the A-BAP group demonstrated statistically and clinically significant improvement from pre- to posttreatment as reflected in the primary outcome measure of depressive symptoms, as well as changes in clinical improvement and in overall functional status ratings made by independent evaluators, blind to treatment condition. All change scores fell within the 95% confidence interval, suggesting that the estimates of change were reliable (McCauley et al., 2015). Although more research on A-BAP is needed to examine efficacy, effectiveness, and predictors of outcome, initial findings suggest that the incorporation of more structured BA strategies could enhance treatment response for depressed adolescents.

In short, BA therapy holds significant potential to expand treatment options for adolescents. In and of itself, BA constitutes an innovative approach to the treatment of depression that is theoretically driven and consistent with the expanding understanding of adolescent development that has emerged from recent findings in cognitive and affective neuroscience. The focus on activation is highly compatible with the developmental needs and abilities of adolescents. Unlike existing therapies that call on sophisticated and higher-order cognitive concepts, BA is an idiographic, behavioral approach that uniquely centers on (1) activation to increase a youth's probability of exposure to naturally rewarding experiences, (2) identification and reduction of barriers to activation, and (3) recognition of avoidance patterns coupled with generation of alternative coping strategies that potentiate the experience of reward for the individual adolescent.

An Overview of the A-BAP

Although this volume presents the A-BAP as a comprehensive intervention, we firmly believe in an individualized approach to treatment. Rather than place the BA approach to treating adolescent depression into a competition with CBT or IPT, we argue the need to draw on strategies that best fit the needs of the individual adolescent. We see the use of BA skills as valuable treatment strategies that can be used as a comprehensive approach or integrated with CBT or IPT strategies as needed.

The A-BAP consists of a series of five modules that can typically be delivered within 12–14 sessions, or as separate "as-needed" components. As noted earlier, detailed session-by-session content is presented in the second section of this volume. There are eight sessions that include a structured didactic component and a set of less structured sessions to be used "as needed" over the course of the intervention. Therapists are encouraged to work collaboratively with the adolescent, take a coaching role, and pace the introduction of skills to match the needs of the adolescent. The program was developed for use with adolescents between ages 12 and 18, and therefore includes materials that are engaging for a younger teen, as well as appropriate for older adolescents approaching adulthood. In an effort to support early engagement and rapid integration of the A-BAP approach, the first two sessions are ideally scheduled in close proximity (e.g., within the same week, if possible). After that, sessions are generally provided once per week, because this schedule seeks to provide optimal care while decreasing the burden of travel time on families and minimizing missed sessions. The sessions are typically 50–60 minutes in length. Therapists can easily modify the session length according to the needs of each adolescent/family and the demands of their practice setting (e.g., school-based work may involve 30-minute encounters, with more limited contact with parents). In most sessions, time is spent with the adolescent alone, followed by a brief intervention with parents. We have suggested some times when the adolescent and parent work together but recognize that this might not work effectively in all settings and with all adolescents, so adaptation may be needed.

The logical progression of A-BAP modules and sessions, outlined in Table 1.1, begins with Module 1, "Getting Started," which typically includes two sessions. In the first session, the overall structure of treatment is reviewed, then therapist and adolescent, with input from the parent(s), work together to establish a shared case conceptualization and an initial set of treatment objectives. The A-BAP model is introduced in this first session and applied to the adolescent's individual circumstances, with activity monitoring being introduced as a "Test It Out" homework assignment (see more details on "Test It Out," p. 14). The second "Getting Started" session is spent mostly with the adolescent, the connection between relationships/activities and mood is presented, and the situation–activity–mood cycle is reviewed. The session ends with a brief meeting with parents to provide some psychoeducation about adolescent depression.

Module 2, "Getting Active," centers on the BA focus and includes material typically covered in two sessions. In Session 3, the concept of goal-directed versus mood-directed behavior is introduced. Additionally, activity–mood monitoring is introduced, building on the concepts of activity monitoring introduced in Session 1. The brief meeting with parents continues the discussion of the parents' experiences parenting a depressed adolescent. The focus on activation for the adolescent is continued in Session 4. Adolescents use a functional-analytic approach to determine what activities work to improve (i.e., "pump you up") their mood and what activities maintain or exacerbate low mood (i.e., "bring you down"), with a secondary focus on identifying the short- and long-term consequences of behavioral choices and how to hold onto a good feeling. In Module 3, "Skill Building" (Sessions 5–8), the A-BAP moves into skills acquisition and reinforcement, with sessions on problem solving, goal setting, and identifying barriers that get in the way of accomplishing goals. Session 8 concludes the module with a focus on strategies for overcoming avoidance that are both introduced and practiced. Module 4, "Practice" (Sessions 9–11), consists of three sessions that are used both to practice and consolidate skills, as needed, according to the adolescent's idiographically determined priorities and goals. Module 5, "Moving Forward," is included to allow time for a review of treatment gains, the adolescent's ongoing goals, and relapse prevention strategies. More specifically, an individualized plan is developed with an eye toward recognizing triggers for depression or other problem behaviors and taking steps to manage mood and avoid escalation of difficulties. This module can be used flexibly over the course of one to three sessions, depending on the needs of the individual adolescent, in order to consolidate treatment gains and terminate therapy.

Although the material in the manual is structured and skills oriented, the intervention is designed to reflect the idiographic nature of BA, such that introduction of skills should be woven into the context of each adolescent's individual experiences. Examples should be drawn from the real-life issues presented by the adolescent. Introduction of a skill may be more general, and the handouts provide hypothetical examples and guidance, but all worksheets include space to add examples specific to the adolescent in treatment. The same principle holds for materials included for parents; a general introduction should be followed by a discussion of examples relevant to the particular family. Throughout the course of treatment, therapists are encouraged to apply concepts flexibly, pulling some skill-building sessions forward and pushing others back, to meet the needs

TABLE 1.1. Structure and Content of the A-BAP

Modules/session	Material covered
Module 1: Getting Started	
Session 1: Introduction to the A-BAP Program	• Review the structure of therapy (confidentiality, roles, use of self-report scale to track symptoms, need for practice outside of sessions). • Review history with both the adolescent and parent for integration into the behavioral activation (BA) model. • Introduce the BA model of depression and treatment. • Using the BA Model and the history provided by adolescent/parent(s), develop a shared case conceptualization. • Introduce activity monitoring.
Session 2: Situation–Activity–Mood Cycle	• Review how relationships and activities impact mood. • Introduce the Situation–Activity–Mood model to the adolescent. • Provide parents with psychoeducation about adolescent depression.
Module 2: Getting Active	
Session 3: Goal-Directed Behavior versus Mood-Directed Behavior	• Introduce the role of activation in mood management—goal-directed versus mood-directed behavior. • Introduce activity–mood monitoring. • Continue to talk with parents about their experiences and concerns as parents of an adolescent who is coping with depression.
Session 4: Introducing Consequences of Behavior	• Introduce functional analysis—the role of reinforcement in maintaining behavior and the importance of evaluating the payoff versus price of behavior choices. • Short-term versus long-term consequences of behavioral choices. • "Pump You Up" and "Bring You Down" activities. • Making the most of good feelings.
Module 3: Skill Building	

Session 5: Problem Solving	• Review the role of stress as a trigger for depression.
	• Introduce problem solving as a way to figure out what to do in stressful situations.
	• Practice using the COPE steps:
	  ○ **C**alm and **c**larify: Calming techniques and problem clarification
	  ○ Generate **O**ptions
	  ○ **P**erform
	  ○ **E**valuate
	• Introduce communication skills to parents and set up communication practice.

Session 6: Goal Setting	• Talk through effective goal setting, the idea of SMART goals. • Introduce the importance of using mini-steps (graded task assignment) to reach a goal. • Set up goal-setting practice for the week. • With parents, walk through ways to show support and set up support monitoring practice.

(continued)

TABLE 1.1. *(continued)*

Modules/session	Material covered
Session 7: Identifying Barriers	• Importance of identifying barriers that get in the way of accomplishing goals. • Internal and external barriers. • Goal-directed versus mood-directed behavior—strategies to overcome barriers. • Goal-setting practice. • Adolescent and parent work together to identify support ideas and set up parent monitoring of their support behavior.
Session 8: Overcoming Avoidance	• Importance of avoidance as a common internal barrier. • Different forms of avoidance—procrastinating, brooding, bursting, and hibernating. • Understanding your Trigger, Response, Avoidance Pattern (TRAP). • Using alternative coping to get back on TRAC. • Review with parent their efforts to practice support.
Module 4: Practice	
Session 9: Putting It All Together	• Review the adolescent's status and identify what he or she wants to focus on for the rest of the therapy sessions. • Review key skills that might be important to helping the adolescent work toward his or her goal—ways to get active, making the most out of good feelings, COPE, goal setting, recognizing barriers, avoidance. • Work with the adolescent to develop an Action Plan to outline priorities, goals, and activities to focus on for the next treatment sessions.
Sessions 10 and 11: Practicing Skills	• Support the adolescent as he or she uses the skills to work on the Action Plan outlined in the previous session. Review the importance of maintaining a focus on working to improve mood/depression.
Module 5: Moving Forward	
Session 12 (or when ending treatment): Relapse Prevention and Saying Good-Bye	• Review and update the Action Plan as needed. • Generate a personal plan for relapse prevention (Doing What Works) to help the adolescent manage triggers and signs of depression. • Review with the adolescent and parent together the adolescent's plans for moving forward and avoiding relapse.

of the particular adolescent and the session-by-session concerns with which he or she presents. It has been our experience, however, that the best way for therapists to become facile with the material and feel comfortable using it flexibly comes with more rigidly applying the protocol a handful of times. Relatedly, it has been the anecdotal report of therapists using the A-BAP that the more facile they become with the material, the more confident they become in taking any of the A-BAP concepts and applying them to the adolescent's unique concerns. Flexibility must also come into play when considering how long to continue working with the adolescent and timing of termination. The A-BAP is written to cover 12 sessions, but getting through the material will differ for each adolescent. Youth seen in settings where only brief contact is possible may still benefit from being introduced to specific A-BAP skills or constructs, whereas other youth may need more time and support to move through the materials. As is true of all therapy, timing of termination must take the individual adolescent's situation and needs into account. For adolescents, even when the material has been covered adequately, terminating treatment in the face of an upcoming, stressful school transition or relationship break-up is frequently not a good idea. In these cases check-in and/or booster sessions to support the youth's success through a difficult transition or to maintain treatment gains can be very useful.

The session-by-session outlines provide prompts for the therapist and suggested dialogue. This material is intended to help bring the specific interventions to life for the therapist and is offered as a guide rather than as a rigid script. Each therapist is advised to adjust the wording to the needs of the adolescent and his or her own style. Although most of the concepts presented in the A-BAP are straightforward, we have found that therapists appreciate the dialogue and prompts as starting points for application with their own clients.

To provide a predictable structure, each session also follows the same general outline. This approach was taken to facilitate clear communication with adolescents about what to expect in therapy, and as a strategy to increase their comfort and sense of partnership with the therapist. Table 1.2 presents an overview of session structure. Each session begins with a "Check-In," which includes asking the adolescent to complete a short self-report scale to monitor depressive symptoms (e.g., Patient Health Questionnaire [PHQ-9]: Richardson et al., 2010; or Short Mood and Feelings Questionnaire [SMFQ]: Messer et al., 1995), followed by a brief review of the adolescent's responses on the scale, the issues the adolescent wants to include on the agenda, and the topics the therapist would like to spend some time on in the session. This provides an opportunity for the adolescent to collaborate with the therapist on finalizing the session agenda, which is often "prepopulated" with material the therapist wants to introduce. It is essential to customize the A-BAP agenda to reflect the primary concerns of each adolescent.

Between-session practice (i.e., "homework") is a core part of the A-BAP and is called "Test It Out." The "Test It Out" component of the A-BAP helps adolescents apply and generalize skills, concepts, and strategies discussed in sessions to practical, everyday problems and situations. Therefore, one of the first agenda items addressed in each session is a review of the "Test It Out" activity generated in the prior session. Following this review, new material is presented, including a clear rationale for each concept or skill introduced, which sets the stage for in-session application or practice of the skill, customized to focus on the concerns raised by the adolescent at the start of the session or in past sessions. A "Test It Out" activity for the coming week is then presented and tailored such that the skill or strategy to be practiced fits the individual adolescent's needs. Even if there is only time to cover part of the material in the session outline, it is important to maintain the overall session structure, with a focus on monitoring symptoms and progress, reviewing practice material, engaging in some in session practice/application, and setting up practice for the upcoming week. The unique needs and concerns of each adolescent must be woven into all skills training and practice exercises.

TABLE 1.2. A-BAP Session Overview

Check-In
- Complete the mood/problem monitoring form.
- Review the monitoring form with the adolescent.
- Check in regarding events/issues that need attention.
- Review/develop a session agenda with the adolescent's input.

Review Practice
- Go over "Test It Out" practice from the last session.

Key Concepts
- Present rationale for work of the session.
- Tie in with the adolescent's individual concerns.
- Tie in with the material/skills covered in prior sessions.

Teach/Skills
- Introduce new material or skills using the adolescent's concerns and examples.

Practice Exercise
- Set up "Test It Out" practice for the coming week.

<u>For time spent with the parent alone</u>

Check-In
- Welcome and invite the parent's questions, observations, concerns.
- Review the session agenda/topic.

Review Practice
- Review "Test It Out" practice if given in the past session.

Teach/Skills
- Present new material.

Practice Exercise
- Set up "Test It Out" practice for the coming week when indicated.

Note. Some sessions also include time for the parent and adolescent to work together and/or time for the parent alone.

Key Intervention Strategies

The A-BAP calls on a set of key components or strategies as the central elements contributing to behavioral changes that in turn lead to improvement in mood and resolution of depression. BA is based on a behavioral model of depression and intervention. Therapists interested in a review of the basics of behavioral psychology might turn to Baum (2005) or Kazdin and Rotella (2013). The essential concepts used in BA include understanding types of reinforcement, particularly response-contingent positive reinforcement, functional analysis, and overcoming avoidance. These are briefly explained on the following page, along with the rationale for the core structural components (monitoring and practice/behavioral rehearsal) and skills included in the program. Finally, the collaborative partnership of the adolescent and care provider, another essential component of the A-BAP, is discussed in the context of techniques for increasing collaboration and enhancing the adolescent's motivation for change.

Reinforcement

For behavioral and cognitive-behavioral therapists, the concept of reinforcement is well understood. However, therapists trained in other therapeutic orientations may be less familiar with the terminology and misunderstandings abound regarding reinforcement. First, reinforcement is not a thing; rather, it is a process. When circumstances are such that the likelihood of a behavior occurring again under similar circumstances is increased, we say that the behavior has been reinforced. Reinforcement can be positive (i.e., something is added to the environment as a consequence of the behavior), or negative (i.e., something is removed). An example of positive reinforcement occurs when a young man goes to gym class, is chosen by his friends to be on their team, then continues to show up on time to class, dressed and ready to participate. We would say that under the circumstances (gym class), the reward he has received from his classmates (being chosen to be on the team) may have reinforced his behavior of reporting on time for class. An example of negative reinforcement occurs in the situation when another boy feels highly anxious about gym class because of his history of little participation in athletic activities. As he approaches the gymnasium for class, he begins to feel a "pit" in his stomach and a mild headache. Instead of going into the gymnasium for class, he goes to the nurse's office and receives a pass to miss class due to illness. He immediately feels less anxiety and the "pit" in his stomach disappears. The next day, he is more likely to have the same sick feelings when he shows up for gym class and may look to be excused from class. We would say that feeling sick has been reinforced because of the reduction (removal) of his anxiety and would expect a subsequent increase in feeling sick and going to the nurse's office.

Behavior can also be shaped through punishment. Positive punishment involves the addition of something following a behavior that decreases the likelihood that the behavior would occur under similar circumstances. A parent tapping a child on the shoulder and giving a stern look when the child is fidgeting in church may extinguish the fidgeting behavior, and we would say the behavior was positively punished. Should the parent take away the child's toy for making noise in church, and the child's noisiness is extinguished, we would say that the behavior was negatively punished.

Lewinsohn (1974) emphasized the impact of response-contingent positive reinforcement in the environments of people who become depressed. Specifically, he proposed that a reduction in response-contingent positive reinforcement may result in depression. Therapists are often confused by the wording and do not fully understand what *response-contingent reinforcement* means. Put very simply, it means that something occurs following the behavior of an adolescent (the response) that reinforces (increases the likelihood to occur again) the behavior. The occurrence of the reinforcing event is contingent on the behavioral response. There are many reasons for reductions in response-contingent positive reinforcement, including the loss of important people in one's environment through death, a move, family separations, or being in an impoverished environment that does not have available rewards. Therapists are also often confused by terms such as *reinforcement*, thinking that positive reinforcement means giving goodies for good behavior, and conflating negative reinforcement and punishment; we hope that we have cleared up these misconceptions. In the A-BAP, while there is never an extensive discussion of reinforcement with the adolescent, a core concept in BA is to work with adolescents to assess how their behavior serves them, and whether it is reinforced or punished; we do this through the process of functional analysis.

Functional Analysis

We refer to a *functional analysis* in BA as a process through which the therapist works with the adolescent to understand how various behavior patterns make sense given the context of the adolescent's life, and also the factors that may maintain depressive behaviors or extinguish positively rewarding behavior. Technically, a functional analysis requires that an experimenter be in control of all variables in the environment in order to understand what contingencies are influencing a behavior. Skinner (1953) himself pointed out that this is not possible when working with human beings in a natural setting, and particularly when working with people who live in the general community as opposed to a controlled environment (e.g., inpatient wards, jails). Nevertheless, less controlled functional analysis is at the heart of BA. Functional analysis is first introduced in Module 2, "Getting Active," and from then on is woven into ongoing discussions with the adolescent about how he or she evaluates options and decides what actions to try. In functional analysis, behavior is not taken at face value because it serves a variety of functions for different people, as well as for the same individual under varied circumstances. For example, "surfing the Internet" as a broad class of behavior can serve many functions. If an adolescent spends 2 hours on the Internet researching dates and important events in ancient Rome, "surfing the Internet" serves an educative function, and in this circumstance, functions as a tool to increase knowledge. That same adolescent may surf the Internet and find friends on Facebook or in other social media. If he or she is doing this during free time, after completing homework and other chores, the behavior functions as a social outlet, and as a pleasurable social activity. Should the circumstances change and the adolescent spends time on Facebook after being told to clean his or her bedroom, the time on the Internet functions as avoidance, procrastination, or willfulness. Finally, should the same adolescent react to teasing at school by feeling blue, self-critical, and unmotivated, and spend time looking on the Internet for stories about famous rock stars or sports figures, lapsing into flights of fancy that he or she will someday be famous and never be teased again, the same activity is functioning as, perhaps, emotional avoidance, numbing, or escape behavior. In addition to attending to functional analysis of the adolescent's behaviors, therapists should teach the adolescent to do a functional analysis of his or her own behavior. This can be done simply by examining the circumstances that occasion particular behaviors and observing the consequence of the behavior. To use less technical language, in the A-BAP, the youth learns how to recognize connections between "situations," his or her behavior, and the consequences, including effects on mood. The consequence can have many components. Emotionally, the behavior may improve or worsen mood; physically, the behavior may bring relief from nervous tension, and there may be consequences that affect others (e.g., parents stop asking the adolescent to do homework) or have other circumstantial consequences (e.g., throwing one's cell phone across a room in a fit of rage might result in the phone breaking). Adolescents can learn to identify the consequence of their behavior and begin to set goals to act in ways that will result in consequences that they desire.

Overcoming Avoidance

Adolescents are also taught about the nature of avoidance, with particular attention to validating the natural tendency to avoid aversive circumstances or feelings. We recognize and acknowledge that avoidance works. On the day of a dreaded examination, staying home sick successfully allows one to avoid taking the test. Sadly, avoidance does not make the dreaded test disappear, and it only postpones the need to take the test, or worse yet, results in a poor grade, which makes an overall bad situation worse. We also can avoid, or try to escape from aversive feelings. In the A-BAP, as in BA in general, we include escape behaviors under the heading of "avoidance" for the sake of simplicity rather than always saying "escape/avoidance." Should one feel sad and depressed, engaging in activities that minimize the feelings or allow one to distract from the feelings (e.g., by spending hours gaming on the Internet) is a logical way to deal with negative emotions. Unfortunately, avoidance tends to keep one stuck in a depressive spiral. One may temporarily escape from or avoid aversive feelings, but one is not actively engaging in activities that could, in the long run, change contexts that may provide the necessary environmental shift that will have antidepressant effects.

The A-BAP teaches the adolescent to recognize when his or her behavior is serving the purpose of avoidance. Once one recognizes that behavior is functionally avoidance behavior, one can experiment with an alternative behavior that is approach- rather than escape-focused. Thus, the adolescent who stayed home sick on examination day may recognize the tendency to avoid studying and take steps to prepare better for a future examination. The adolescent who spends hours gaming to escape from or avoid aversive feelings may call a trusted friend and seek social support that leads to a sense of being connected and cared for, and therefore less depressed.

Key Structural Elements

Monitoring

There is growing evidence of the importance and utility of routine monitoring of symptom change in response to treatment (Bickman, Kelley, Breda, de Andrade, & Riemer, 2011; Goodman, McKay, & DePhilippis, 2013; Lyon, Borntrager, Nakamura, & Higa-McMillan, 2013). Routine progress or symptom monitoring has been associated with "higher rates of reliable and significant symptom change" in studies of adults, college students (Lambert et al., 2002; Miller, Sorensen, Selzer, & Brigham, 2006), and youth (Bickman et al., 2011). Monitoring symptom or behavioral change provides valuable feedback to the therapist, adolescent, and parent about progress being made or the need to consider revisions to the treatment approach. In addition progress or symptom monitoring has been demonstrated to improve communication between care providers and clients (Carlier et al., 2012). For these reasons, regular symptom monitoring has been included in the A-BAP. Collaborative and routine review of the symptoms or behaviors that are the target of treatment facilitates discussion of what symptoms/problems are most troublesome to the adolescent and in turn guides the focus of care. This process also ensures that the adolescent and therapist understand the kinds of behavior change toward which they are working. This in turn makes the therapy process more transparent and enhances the collaborative nature of the adolescent–therapist relationship. Monitoring also provides a way to track the status of critical areas in addition to the emergence of new problems, such as increases in suicidality through a weekly review of high-risk behaviors. Monitoring additional targets, such as self-harming behavior, anxiety, or poor school attendance, may be useful with some adolescents and can be easily incorporated as long as assessments are brief and used judiciously so as not to overburden the adolescent or cause confusion regarding treatment goals.

Behavior Rehearsal/Practice

Throughout the history of behavioral skills training, the importance of having clients practice or rehearse behavior has been emphasized. The A-BAP program encourages rehearsal and practice of all new behavior. Practice may occur during the session, and it most certainly occurs between sessions through encouragement and administration of "Test It Out" activities. There is evidence that homework adherence is a critical component of CBT for adults (Kazantzis, Whittington, & Dattilio, 2010), as well as CBT for adolescent depression (Clarke et al., 1992; Gaynor, Lawrence, & Nelson-Gray, 2006). We consider behavior rehearsal to be important for two reasons: First, it allows the therapist and adolescent to assess the adolescent's skill level during implementation of new strategies; second, it serves as an experiment for the adolescent to test different strategies to determine what is useful. We do not expect adolescents to take our word that changing their behavior will change their mood, so we ask them to try out new behaviors using the "Test-It-Out" practice and pay attention to or observe the impact on mood. As part of this, we emphasize that even a small change in mood for a brief moment in time can be a building block for more significant change overtime.

Skill Building

The A-BAP includes a focus on the introduction and practice of a set of concepts, skills, and strategies that are central to the BA model, such as functional analysis and overcoming avoidance, as discussed earlier. Problem solving and goal setting were included in the skill-building component, because these skills were significantly associated with improved response in prior studies of the treatment of depression in adolescents (Kennard et al., 2009); furthermore, these skills provide the adolescent with clear strategies or a set of steps to take when approaching a wide variety of problems and can be used to guide resolution of social (peer pressure, bullying), communication (family, teacher, peer conflicts), and emotion regulation (anger, impulsivity, anxiety) issues, thus covering broadly the bases of challenging situations faced by most youth.

Involvement of Parents in the A-BAP

The A-BAP actively includes parents as key collaborators in the treatment process. Parents play a unique role in three specific ways that may influence a course of the A-BAP. First, parents hold decision-making authority about many of the adolescent's activities that may be considered during A-BAP sessions. Similarly, they hold access to practical resources such as transportation that may influence an adolescent's ability to do certain activities. This may be even more the case among younger adolescents, who may not yet be allowed to take public transportation independently and cannot drive for themselves. It is essential to engage parents as collaborators in the selection and utilization of activities to support their adolescent. Second, parents may be part of the communication and interaction cycles with the adolescent that serve to maintain the adolescent's depression over time. Thus, engaging parents in understanding and modifying these cycles is also important. For these reasons, the A-BAP conceptualizes treatment as a team-based approach in which each member (therapist, parent, and adolescent) plays a critical and unique role. Third, adolescents may underplay or ineffectively communicate the level of distress they experience, and it is important to have multiple sources for assessing how treatment is working. Therefore, regular contact and teamwork with the parent(s), as well as using both parent and adolescent ratings of the adolescent's symptoms if feasible, is important for ongoing assessment and planning.

The A-BAP engages parents early in treatment with psychoeducation about adolescent depression and the BA model. Later sessions also include education about specific strategies to improve communication with adolescents and concrete actions to support adolescents' efforts to reach treatment goals. Parents are asked to participate in the majority of sessions, including spending time with the therapist and adolescent together, as well as spending parts of sessions alone with the therapist. Having the adolescent and parent together in a session is feasible with only some adolescents/families, so this is, of course, optional. Parents are encouraged to support adolescents practicing skills outside of sessions and, at times, they too are given "Test It Out" activities to complete between sessions.

Involvement of family members helps others in the home to understand the behavioral model of depression and to be aware of the strategies that the adolescent will be using to engage in his or her life and break out of the depressive cycle. For example, adolescents are taught about effective goal setting and identifying barriers to goals. During this discussion, the therapist inquires about how the adolescent's parent may facilitate or interfere with accomplishing a goal or a mini-step within a given goal. If an adolescent identifies a parent's behavior as creating a barrier toward the goal, the therapist and adolescent may consider how best to engage the parent in a discussion about how to resolve this problem. The parent joins the session and together they problem-solve about how the parent can best support the adolescent's goal. After spending time all together, there is time for the therapist and parent to meet alone, without the adolescent. This provides the therapist and parent a chance to discuss any important concerns or collateral information that may be further complicating the adolescent's ability to move toward a goal. This time also may involve the therapist providing psychoeducation about the need for many parents to alter their expectations of a depressed adolescent or reframing how they think about "support," such that they are facilitating their adolescent's efforts to increase and change behaviors.

The amount of personal information about the adolescent that is shared with the parent or family member in individual contacts must be negotiated with the adolescent in treatment, as issues of confidentiality need to be considered, and maintaining a trusting and collaborative relationship is important. Therapists can involve the parents in general discussions of BA, teach them skills for listening to their adolescent, and help them learn new ways to be supportive without divulging personal information that the adolescent may not wish to have disclosed. Parents also can receive support for the challenges of raising an adolescent and the particular difficulties of dealing with a depressed adolescent. More specifically, therapists can help parents reframe the adolescent's irritability, which is sometimes extreme, as a function of his or her depression. This in turn can help parents put in perspective what their teen is going through and, instead of becoming punitive in the face of perceived disrespect, take a more supportive stance. Parents can also sometimes fall into extreme categories, from those who are mostly uninvolved with their child's life to those who micromanage their son or daughter. It is understandable, particularly in the case of suicidal adolescents, that a parent's concern can result in overprotection that is experienced as intrusive by the adolescent. Therefore, it is essential that therapists establish a collaborative environment in which to negotiate levels of involvement that are tolerable, practical, and helpful for all involved.

Collaborating with the Adolescent and Enhancing Motivation for Change

Collaboration between the therapist and the adolescent is at the heart of the treatment. In relation to the adolescent, the A-BAP therapist is more like a "coach" than a medical expert. The coach serves as a collaborative partner who teaches and supports the adolescent in learning and engaging in the BA approach. Coaches work with athletes to discuss, teach, and support a plan for engaging in a sport or athletic endeavor, but it is the athlete who must undertake the play. This is true in the A-BAP as well. The therapist, as a coach, instructs the adolescent in the concepts that are central to treatment, and works with the adolescent to develop a plan that the adolescent will test out by implementing it between sessions. Just as a coach and athlete review the execution of a play in a sport, the A-BAP therapist and the adolescent (or parent) debrief the activities that have occurred between sessions, make necessary adjustments, and collaborate on any changes that will be attempted over the following week. Similar "debriefing" occurs with parents when they practice with "Test It Out" exercises between sessions. Over the course of treatment, the therapist shares responsibility with the adolescent for the work, assuming that the adolescent will take greater responsibility over time, thereby promoting the adolescent's sense of self-efficacy for doing the work.

Activating depressed adolescents is a challenging task. The symptoms of depression often include lack of motivation, low mood, inertia, and fatigue. Engaging in usual activities may have become both psychologically and physically more difficult than it was prior to the onset of depression. Lack of motivation may, in part, reflect the adolescent's diminished capacity to experience previously enjoyable activities as rewarding, and may require careful attention to enhancement of motivation to initiate behaviors. To this end, motivational strategies are used throughout the course of the A-BAP (Naar-King & Suarez, 2011). The BA model assumes that behavioral patterns persist because they are reinforced. Thus, adolescents may engage in very reinforcing behaviors that in the long run maintain their depression. It is incumbent upon the therapist to use strategies that motivate the adolescent to change such behaviors, so that new, antidepressant behaviors have the possibility of being reinforced in the environment. The A-BAP draws on some of the motivational techniques developed as part of the Motivational Interviewing (MI) treatment approach (Miller & Rollnick, 2002). *Evocation*, or recognition of the adolescent as the expert, and *collaboration* to elicit the adolescent's understanding of intervention strategies, and particularly the ways in which the strategies are relevant to the adolescent's situation are two MI-based principles the A-BAP employs.

Although there is clearly a didactic component to many of the A-BAP sessions, they are intended to be presented by therapists who, again, draw on motivational principles to engage the adolescent effectively (Naar-King & Suarez, 2011). This includes demonstrating optimal *empathy* and understanding of the adolescent's life context and potential struggles. The therapist also is encouraged to use the core MI communication approach using *open-ended questions*, *affirmations*, *reflective listening*, and *summaries* to clarify the "take-home messages" in order to enhance motivation. For example, when talking with an adolescent about skipping class to avoid feelings of anxiety about math, the therapist asks in an open-ended, neutral fashion about any disadvantages of this approach, points out how it makes sense given how uncomfortable the adolescent feels in class, summarizes what he or she is hearing, checks with the adolescent to be sure he or she is on track, and ends each encounter with a brief summary of what they have learned together and a review of the next steps. In this collaborative approach, therapists are encouraged to "check-in" frequently with the adolescent, as well as his or her parents, to assess the goodness of fit of specific strategies being implemented. Adolescents and families are more likely to follow through if they agree that the treatment strategies are appropriate in their particular situation. Therefore it is important that the A-BAP therapist makes every effort to assure that the behavioral conceptualization of depression, presented in their BA working model, is relevant to the adolescent and family. There is no better way of knowing whether one is on the mark than to check-in with the adolescent directly.

Summary

The A-BAP is designed to increase systematically the adolescent's engagement in activities so as to alter his or her avoidance patterns, and to help him or her learn and practice skills for problem solving and for managing difficult emotions. The program emphasizes reducing problematic behaviors, as well as increasing positive behaviors. Therapists may follow the program as written, keeping each session in the order presented in the manual. However, the program was intended to allow enough flexibility that therapists can skip topics that may be less relevant to a particular adolescent. If the therapist determines that following a different sequence of sessions makes more sense given an adolescent's needs, he or she needs to be mindful that the "Test It Out" homework exercises are consistent between sessions assuring that this essential ingredient of therapy is not overlooked. Therapists are strongly encouraged, if possible, given the work setting, to include parents or at least provide them with materials that teach about adolescent depression and include tips for supporting their adolescent. Helping parents understand their adolescent's depression and learn strategies to improve their communication and support can be essential to a successful therapeutic outcome in some cases.

Throughout treatment the therapist should keep in mind that the ultimate goal is transfer of training into the adolescent's real life, and generalization of in-session content to the adolescent's daily life is important from the beginning of treatment onward. The final sessions are meant to be flexible in terms of number, because some adolescents need more time and support to overcome their depression, and the timing of important life transitions, such as starting a new school or breaking off a relationship, needs to be considered when moving toward the conclusion of therapy. Related to this, therapists can schedule maintenance or "check-in" sessions periodically, following completion of the program, as a way to ensure that the adolescent maintains treatment gains and is not falling back into the trap of avoidance behaviors in the face of life transitions and stressors.

CHAPTER 2

Assessment, Case Conceptualization, and Treatment Planning

Assessment, case conceptualization, and treatment planning are the cornerstones of any intervention program, and it is no different with regard to the A-BAP. As such, each is reviewed and discussed here. More specifically, we begin this chapter with a brief discussion of which depressed youth are appropriate for a BA approach and which are not. This is followed by a brief overview of assessment and case conceptualization issues, with case examples and their conceptualization within the BA model. We close the chapter with a discussion of how assessment and case conceptualization information is incorporated into an A-BAP treatment plan.

Who Is and Is Not an Appropriate Youth for the BA Approach

Several questions come into play with regard to deciphering who is and who is not an appropriate candidate for the A-BAP. The first question centers on whether a youth must have a "pure" depression to benefit from BA treatment. Although adolescents in our randomized trial all had a primary diagnosis of a depressive disorder (e.g., major depression, dysthymia, unspecified depressive disorder), we believe that they were representative of youth seen in most "real-life" clinical settings and a true clinical sample, in that very few had a "pure" depression. More specifically, we worked with youth with co-occurring anxiety, mild externalizing symptoms, and low average intelligence (e.g., IQ between 70 and 85). Although we did not have the sample size to support analyses on differential outcomes for these various subgroups, our anecdotal experience with these youth suggested that the A-BAP approach was effective and helpful even in the presence of these co-occurring symptoms. Even though we purposefully ruled out youth who struggled with subthreshold depressive symptoms, we believe that the A-BAP also could have been helpful and effective with this population.

The second question centers on whether the A-BAP can be beneficial for depressed youth with suicidality. Although chronic and severe forms of suicidality may be better addressed through other forms of treatment (see below), mild to moderate levels of suicidality associated with depression can be addressed, more than adequately, using the A-BAP. Just as therapists should track changes in depressive symptoms, they should also track changes in suicidal thoughts, feelings, and behaviors. Such symptoms then become targets of treatment, with special attention paid to how aspects of the adolescent's environment lead to increases or decreases in suicidal ideation. Additionally, because it is not uncommon for reports of suicidality to emerge as treatment for depression progresses, we recommend that in addition to assessing suicidality at the outset, it is important to monitor this on an ongoing basis for all youth.

The third question centers on whether there are diagnoses for which the A-BAP would not be the treatment model of choice. The answer to this is a resounding "yes." The last decade has seen significant advances in the development of effective interventions for many child and adolescent psychiatric and behavioral disorders (Weisz, Jensen-Doss, & Hawley, 2006), and the A-BAP, outlined here, has been specifically designed to treat adolescent depression. Therefore, when a specific, well-supported treatment is available, it is best to use the treatment designed and tested for specific problems, such as Barkley's (2005) approach for management of attention-deficit/hyperactivity disorder (ADHD). Although the use of a BA approach with adolescents appears to be a very promising alternative or adjunct to CBT and IPT, data supporting its utility with a wide range of other forms of severe psychopathology do not exist. More specifically, the A-BAP is not a treatment for youth with psychosis or bipolar disorder. Although some aspects of BA could conceivably be helpful and might be incorporated into care, there are other promising treatments for these youth, including interpersonal and social rhythm therapy for adolescents (IPSRT-A; Hlastala, Kotler, McClellan, & McCauley, 2010) with bipolar disorder. Likewise, the A-BAP would not be the treatment of choice for youth with a primary diagnosis of substance abuse or dependence, significant conduct difficulties and disruptive behavior, significant intellectual disabilities, autism spectrum disorders, and more serious suicidality and/or chronic self-harm associated with marked emotional dysregulation. Investigators (e.g., Linehan, McCauley, Berk, & Asarnow, 2012) are currently studying the appropriateness of using a dialectical behavior therapy (DBT; Linehan, 1993) model with chronically suicidal/self-harming youth—an approach that makes sense clinically given DBT's focus on emotion regulation and distress tolerance skills. Also, individuals whose functioning is primarily impaired by obsessive–compulsive disorder or posttraumatic stress symptoms would likely be better served by exposure and response prevention (ERP; Foa & Kozak, 1986; Piacentini, March, & Franklin, 2006) and trauma-focused cognitive-behavioral therapy (TF-CBT; Cohen, Mannarino, & Deblinger, 2006) respectively. BA strategies may prove helpful in working with youth who present with these clinical problems but, particularly at this early stage of BA studies, use of these strategies should only be seen as a way to augment or facilitate delivery of interventions with well-established efficacy.

Assessment

A-BAP treatment planning hinges on careful attention to case conceptualization based on use of a multitrait, multimethod (MTMM) assessment (Campbell & Fiske, 1959) whenever possible. Therapists need to assess for and understand the presence of depressive symptoms and the context in which they occur, as well as the presence of co-occurring symptoms and the context in which they occur, because presence of other problems may indicate that another treatment approach would be more appropriate. Furthermore, symptoms alone are not the only focus of BA, and therapists must attend to impairment in functioning in all areas of the adolescent's life. Although using an MTMM approach to assessment can be somewhat time-consuming, the use of such an approach enhances the therapist's understanding of the presenting difficulties, which in turn allows him or her to develop a comprehensive case formulation that can then be used to individualize and guide treatment over time. True to the MTMM approach, this case formulation is best accomplished when therapists collect information across a variety of domains (multitrait), utilizing a range of measurement tools (e.g., questionnaires, clinical interviews) and informants (e.g., adolescent, parent, teacher, other) (multi-method). The following section outlines the scope of information obtained with an MTMM assessment approach that can optimally inform the A-BAP case conceptualization.

Scope of Differential Diagnosis and Co-Occurring Disorders

In recent years, diagnostic clarification has shifted from a focus on establishing categorical diagnoses to integrating and emphasizing a dimensional consideration of symptoms (American Psychiatric Association, 2013; Helzer, Kraemer, & Krueger, 2006; Kraemer, 2007). This shift reflects our understanding that individuals evidence varying levels of severity within disorders and frequently evidence symptoms across diagnostic categories. Measuring symptoms dimensionally allows therapists to capture the acuity of symptoms, as well as the presence of important co-occurring disorders that could affect treatment selection and implementation. Research demonstrates that between 40 and 70% of children/adolescents with major depressive disorder (MDD) have at least one co-occurring psychiatric diagnosis, and between 20 and 50% of children/adolescents with MDD have two or more psychiatric diagnoses (Birmaher, Ryan, Williamson, Brent, & Kaufman, 1996). Without careful assessment using a multitrait approach, co-occurring problems could go undetected and in turn impact treatment response and outcome. For the purposes of the A-BAP, taking this type of broad, dimensional approach ensures that all relevant symptoms are assessed. For example, depressive and anxious symptoms often go hand in hand. If assessment indicates that, in addition to symptoms of depression, an adolescent also endorses worry and social anxiety, it would be important to gain a thorough understanding of how these symptoms manifest and affect the adolescent's mood and functioning. A therapist working with an adolescent with social anxiety should be careful to assess how this will affect practice or "Test It Out" tasks and subsequently calibrate the intervention appropriately. For example, the therapist may provide focused psychoeducation on how social anxiety can function as an internal barrier to completing mini-steps toward a goal and identify ways to manage this barrier. Additionally, some disorders, such as disruptive behavior disorders, are considered "gateway" disorders to adolescent depression (Burke, Loeber, Lahey, & Rathouz, 2005). A comprehensive assessment that includes both symptom clusters allows the therapist to intervene more effectively. If a youth's depression is secondary to the negative consequences of conduct problems, it is important to work with the adolescent to identify, schedule, and reinforce healthy pleasant activities. Clarification of the various factors, including life circumstances and co-occurring symptoms that may be triggering or sustaining depressive or dysfunctional behavior, is central to the A-BAP because this is what guides the development of strategies to establish alternate reinforcing behaviors.

Informant Variability

The importance of gathering data regarding symptoms and levels of impairment from various informants, while useful in planning any therapeutic treatment plan, is particularly important in the A-BAP. Collecting information on the adolescent's presentation from both the adolescent and his or her parent(s) is, of course, essential. Failure to do so will inevitably leave a therapist unaware of important aspects of the adolescent's story and without a complete picture of his or her symptom presentation. More specifically, symptom reports often differ between parents and youth (Edelbrock, Costello, Dulcan, Conover, & Kalas, 1986), and parents and youth do not always agree that a problem exists. While parents tend to focus more on externalizing behaviors and what they can see, adolescents may focus more on their own internal experience and minimize what their parents find alarming. Data from both informants are particularly critical within the A-BAP, because of the need for detailed understanding of what factors might be reinforcing, perhaps inadvertently, the adolescent's depressive behaviors. Although it is often tempting to try to save time by meeting with parents and youth together, we suggest that at least some portion of the clinical interview involve youth and the parents alone. Not only does this allow the therapist an opportunity to establish the adolescent as the primary focus of care, but it further allows each party individual time with the therapist. Some adolescents are highly reluctant to share aspects of their symptoms/experiences with their parents in the room. Likewise parents often have information they wish to share without the adolescent present. Failure to interview parents and youth separately can lend itself to the loss of important information. That said, it is equally important to be clear with each party what will be shared and what will be kept confidential. More specifically, parents need to know that the adolescent will be kept informed of all contact with the parent and the general theme of the contact (e.g., "Your mom called me earlier this week because she was worried about your school attendance"), but that the reverse is not true and that what adolescents say is confidential within the normal limits (e.g., danger to self, danger to other, abuse). In formulating a treatment plan within the A-BAP model, it is important to understand, for instance, how both the adolescent and his or her parent(s) perceive his or her limited activities with friends. More specifically, is this troublesome to the adolescent and secondary to low mood and social withdrawal or rewarding because of unlimited access to Internet games and exploration? Is it a worry to parents or secondary to parents' inability to provide transportation or needed funding, or their preference for the adolescent to be home, part of family activities, or caring for siblings? Information from multiple informants, including school personnel, can also often offer important insights into an adolescent's difficulties that add to the case conceptualization and may help to identify potential targets for activation or areas in which avoidance is particularly significant.

Development

The A-BAP depends on understanding the context of an adolescent's behavior; therefore, it is also important to consider the adolescent's developmental status. Because adolescents are constantly growing and experiencing change—physically, cognitively, emotionally, and socially—therapists need to decipher whether their symptoms are normative or pathological, and whether these symptoms represent transient developmental phenomena or something more enduring and serious. It is not enough to make assumptions about maturity based on the age of the youth. As we discussed in Chapter 1, significant neurocognitive development occurs during adolescence. We have learned that the maturation of response inhibition, problem solving, and long-term planning skills emerges gradually over the course of adolescence and young adulthood (Somerville et al., 2010; Steinberg et al., 2006). Therefore, careful attention should be given to assessing the ability of the adolescent, particularly the young adolescent, who may present as physically mature and worldly, to observe and alter behavioral response patterns. In the A-BAP, this information would inform the focus and pacing of treatment. The less cognitively mature adolescent may benefit from more time and attention on core concepts and structuring of "Test It Out" activities, while the more mature adolescent may be able to move more quickly into functional analyses of his or her avoidance behaviors. Similarly, the less cognitively mature adolescent may require more parental involvement for scheduling and planning, while the more mature adolescent may manage this effectively on his or her own.

A change in sleep habits is another example of an important developmental factor to assess. With puberty, adolescents have an increased physiological need for sleep but at the same time experience a shift in natural sleep–wake cycles that leads to a preference for going to sleep later in the day and having more difficulty rising early in the morning (Carskadon, 2002). Careful assessment of bedtime habits and sleep changes in adolescents, including attention to late night phone and Internet activity, and parental education about these naturally occurring changes in sleep patterns, allows a therapist to discern whether this would be best thought of as part of natural biological development or a symptom of depression.

Another developmental challenge involves the common transition from children seeing their parents as their most important relationship to seeing their peers and friends as primary. This shift may be experienced by parents as concerning if they perceive their adolescent to be withdrawing or becoming increasingly irritable and potentially depressed. Once again, in the context of assessing an adolescent for depression, a therapist would pay attention to how the adolescent's relationships and ability to seek and secure social support is affecting his or her functioning and would be able to get a sense of whether this shift was part of normative development or reflective of problems with depression.

With all symptoms and behavioral changes, whether they are related to development or not, it is also important to try to discern whether the adolescent demonstrates a noticeable change from his or her usual self. This may be better assessed by the parent; however, it is important to get input from all informants.

Tools for Symptom Assessment

Many tools exist for assessing symptoms and behavioral patterns (for a comprehensive review, see Klein, Dougherty, & Olino, 2005). While all therapists tend to have their favorite tools, we recommend that they focus on tools that allow them to (1) understand the timing of the patient's symptoms and behaviors (e.g., depression in context; see below); (2) make a systematic diagnosis of depression and rule out co-occurring disorders that may suggest an alternative treatment (e.g., a comprehensive clinical interview that is supplemented by a broad-based self-report and caregiver report of symptoms, such as the Youth Self-Report Form [YSR] and the Child Behavior Checklist [CBCL; Achenbach, 2009]); and (3) track session by session changes in depressive symptoms and suicidality (e.g., SMFQ: Angold et al., 1995; PHQ-9: Richardson et al., 2010). In assessing the cases outlined below, assessment tools included the SMFQ (Angold et al., 1995; clinical cutoff score of 11), the Suicide Ideation Questionnaire (SIQ; Reynolds, 1987; clinical cutoff of 89th percentile), the YSR (clinical cutoff *T*-score of 70), and the CBCL (Achenbach, 2009; clinical cutoff *T*-score of 70).

Understanding Depression in Context

Throughout both assessment and treatment, it is critical to collect information about contextual factors in the adolescent's life. Such factors may include cultural issues, general adversity and stressors (both significant life events and daily hassles), as well as the role of school, social interactions, and interpersonal relationships with peers, family, and other important individuals (e.g., teachers, coaches, friends' parents). Given the importance of the ongoing functional analysis of factors that affect mood, activation, and avoidance, taking time to elucidate contextual factors is important for case conceptualization and also provides another opportunity to build rapport. Much of this data collection happens informally during the session; however, we recommend that therapists also utilize tools that support the more systematic tracking of such data. We have included a tool that we developed, a Depression Timeline (see Figure 2.1), as it guides the therapist to understand the timeline of the adolescent's mood, symptoms, stressors, relationships, and the effect of school. While it is important to determine the adolescent's diagnostic profile, it is also important to understand the timeline by which his or her symptoms emerged, the context in which the symptoms emerged, factors/stressors linked to the emergence of such symptoms, and the level of impairment associated with symptoms at various points in time. The completion of a Depression Timeline provides an approach to gathering and putting this information together. More specifically, the therapist can use it as a tool to

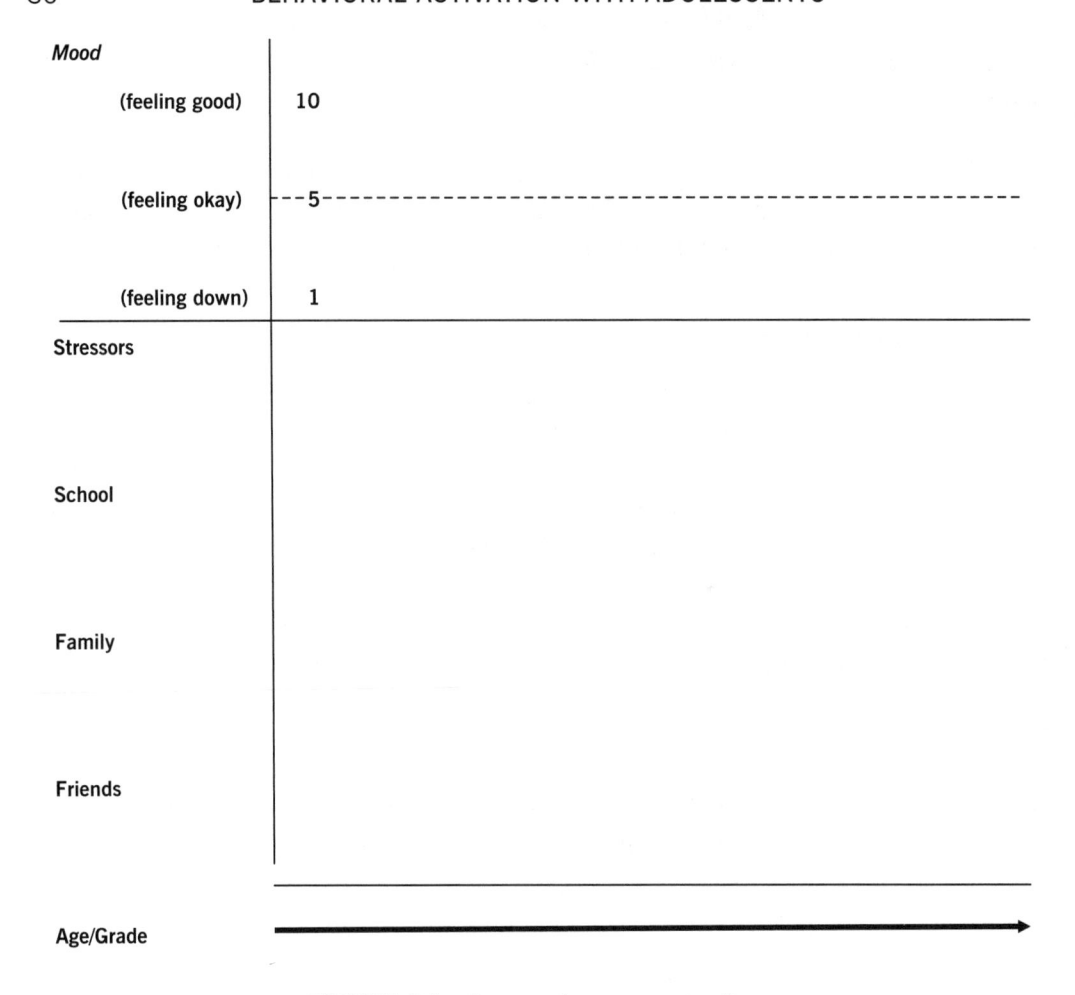

```
Mood
        (feeling good)     10

        (feeling okay)  ---5----------------------------------------------

        (feeling down)      1

Stressors


School


Family


Friends


Age/Grade          ──────────────────────────────▶
```

FIGURE 2.1. Current depression timeline.

guide an interview of the adolescent and his or her parents, in an open-ended fashion, to understand the timing of different events, situations, and symptoms in the adolescent's life and gain clarification on the adolescent's history. Through the use of a timeline, a therapist can more readily establish the onset and offset of symptoms, stressors, and associated impairments to aid in the selection of other assessment tools and more readily focus the diagnostic assessment. The timeline format is shown in Figure 2.1.

Case Conceptualization

Regardless of the assessment battery utilized, the therapist's job is to put the data together in a clear and coherent case conceptualization that is idiographic in nature and leads to an individualized application of the BA model to the unique circumstances in the adolescent's life. The BA model as presented in Chapter 1, Figure 1.1, provides a useful guide for case conceptualization and planning.

A number of factors, both predisposing (e.g., genetics and a family history of depression) and precipitating (e.g., academic stress, peer conflict), may contribute to the emergence of depressive symptoms in youth. The BA model of depression highlights the notion that the circumstances of the depressed youth's situation, that is, the presence of negative experiences or stressors and the lack of rewarding experiences, contributes to a range of symptoms such as sadness, fatigue, irritability, anhedonia, feelings of worthlessness, and perhaps even feelings of suicidality. The natural human response to such symptoms is to hunker down, isolate, sleep, skip school and/or schoolwork, and blend into the woodwork. Such behavior creates a series of negative consequences that in turn form a negative feedback loop leading to worsening symptoms (e.g., when an adolescent withdraws from friends and school, friends stop calling, grades fall, and parents get on the youth's case). This, in turn, lends itself to the feeling that life is even less rewarding and life circumstances are worsening, and the vicious cycle of depression continues. Within the BA framework, the key is to break the negative feedback loop by doing something different in the face of depressive symptoms—typically, something that connects the adolescent to positive and rewarding experiences, thus helping him or her to reengage in the world rather than further isolating. This, in turn, typically limits the potential for further negative consequences.

Below are four case examples that demonstrate the A-BAP case conceptualization, followed by a discussion of how this information informs treatment planning.

Vignette 1

Peter is a 13-year-old boy who lives with his biological parents and younger brother. Peter has a history of ADHD that began in kindergarten but has been well managed with stimulant medication over the years. Peter's younger brother struggles with mild cognitive delays and some significant behavioral difficulties that require a great deal of time and attention from their parents. Given his brother's difficulties, Peter's needs have unintentionally come second. According to his parents, Peter has gradually become increasingly focused on "keeping the peace" around his brother, letting him have his way, and generally avoiding any interaction with his brother that he fears will lead to an argument or tantrum. Peter's parents are keenly aware of this, attempt to spend time with Peter alone, and frequently give him the opportunity to discuss his concerns and not put his brother's needs before his own. But, like many boys his age, Peter is very uncomfortable talking about emotions. Despite these attempts, Peter's parents have noticed that he has been spending more time alone in his room and has become more socially isolated—no longer inviting friends to the house or accepting invitations to spend time with friends outside of school. In addition, by their report, Peter appears sad, struggles with irritability, has lost interest in some of his usual activities, is spending more time sleeping, has significant difficulty concentrating on his schoolwork, and makes occasional comments about being worthless. Both of Peter's parents have tried to talk with Peter about their observations, and each attempt is met with "I am fine" and "Nothing is bothering me." A timeline summarizing Peter's history is outlined in Figure 2.2.

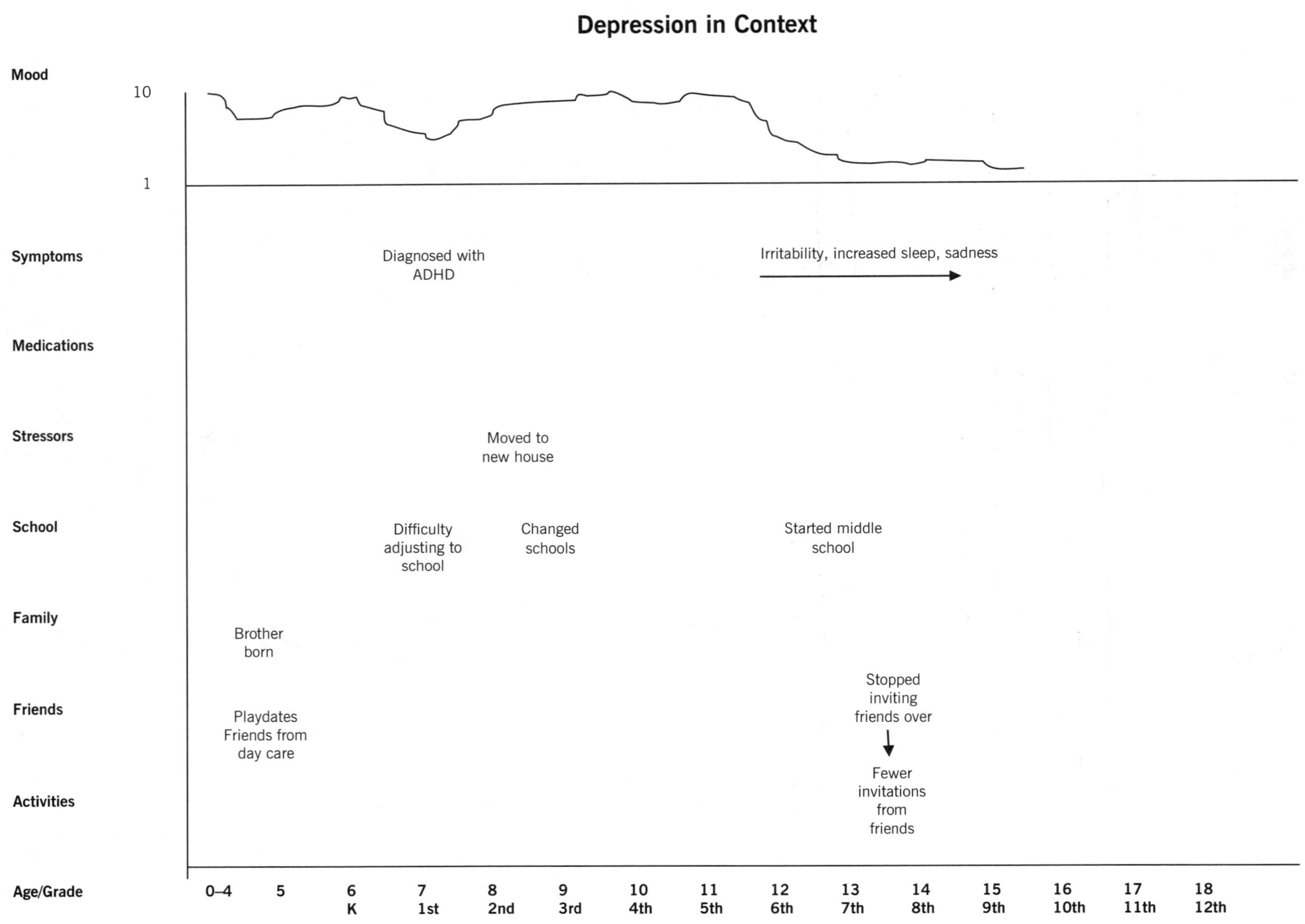

FIGURE 2.2. Completed timeline for Peter.

Peter's Assessment Data

Peter provides an excellent example of why it is important to gather collateral data from parents, or others, whenever possible. Upon intake, Peter denied symptoms of depression while his parents endorsed a range of symptoms that led to a diagnosis of unspecified depressive disorder. This differential pattern of symptom endorsement, with Peter reporting few symptoms and parents endorsing many symptoms, was also found in questionnaire data. More specifically, while Peter denied difficulties with depression on the SMFQ, with a total score of 0, his parents' score was 18, suggesting the presence of a number of significant depressive symptoms. Moreover Peter's very low score raised doubts about the validity of his responses. Similarly, while Peter endorsed few symptoms of anxiety and depression on the YSR (Anxious–Depressed T-score = 50), his parents noted significant concerns (Anxious–Depressed T-score = 76). While both Peter and his parents agreed that suicidality, as well as other psychiatric symptoms, were not of major concern via both interview and questionnaire data (e.g., SIQ at the 50th percentile, YSR Externalizing T-score = 43, and CBCL Externalizing T-score = 54), the point remains that they had significantly different perceptions with regard to symptoms of depression. This is where clinical judgment played a central role. Peter presented as a young adolescent who is clearly uncomfortable talking about emotion, and despite significant behavioral indicators of depression on mental status examination (e.g., he appeared sad, teared up at times, his rate of speech and movement was somewhat slow), Peter held strongly to the idea that "nothing is wrong." These behavioral observations, in addition to the significant discrepancy in Peter's self-report and that of his parents with regard to his symptomatology, allowed the therapist to feel comfortable in weighing parental report over self-report and making the recommendation to begin a course of treatment focused on activation.

Peter's Case Conceptualization

The case conceptualization begins with an understanding of the circumstances of Peter's life that have ultimately contributed to his subjective experience of sadness and irritability, his withdrawal from friends, and difficulties concentrating in school. The A-BAP case conceptualization for Peter is depicted within the BA model in Figure 2.3. Not only are his brother's behavioral difficulties annoying to him but they also require a great deal of time on the part of his parents, with the end result of Peter getting the "short end of the stick" when it comes to attention. In fact, Peter has become so focused on trying not to make matters worse that he has placed his brother's needs before his own. Peter has tried to maintain a profile of invisibility in his family, and the rewards he once enjoyed (e.g., positive interactions with his brother, attention from his parents) have been put to the wayside (see "Life Circumstances" in Figure 2.3). Peter's subjective experience of his "life circumstances" has manifested in a number of symptoms (see "How do you feel?" in Figure 2.3), including sadness, irritability, worthlessness, and poor concentration, which are abundantly apparent to others, but which Peter himself does not describe. Peter's response to his depressive feelings (see "What do you do?" in Figure 2.3) and attempts to

```
┌─────────────────┐      ┌─────────────────┐      ┌─────────────────┐
│ Life Circumstances:│      │ How do you feel?:│      │ What do you do?:│
│ Stress related to │ ───► │ Sadness, irritability,│ ───► │ Social isolation, failure to│
│ brother's difficulties│      │ worthlessness, poor│      │ complete schoolwork,│
│ Lack of attention │      │ concentration    │      │ increased sleep │
│ from parents      │      │                  │      │                 │
└─────────────────┘      └─────────────────┘      └─────────────────┘
```

Reinforce idea → & feed into depressive symptoms

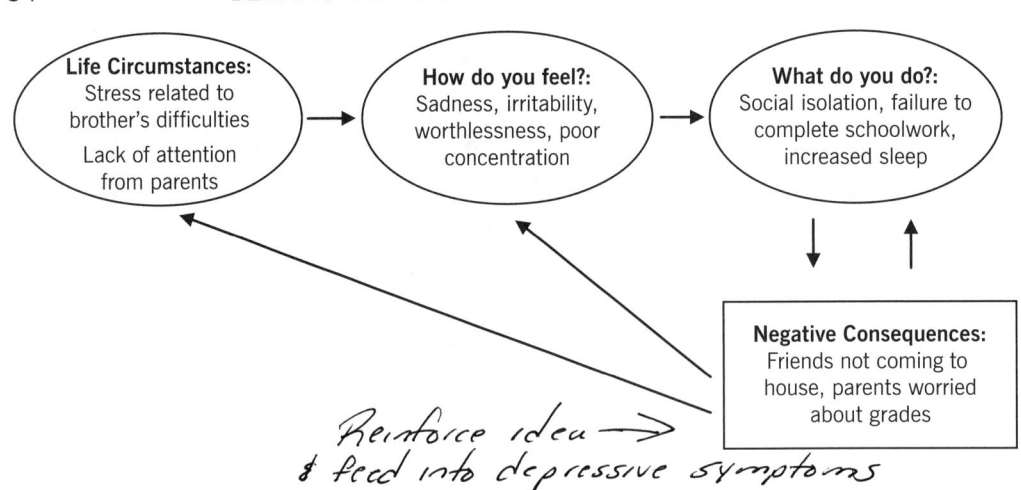

FIGURE 2.3. Peter's case conceptualization within the BA model.

manage his symptoms have inadvertently resulted in a range of behaviors that are avoidant in nature and have limited his connection with the world around him (e.g., social isolation, a failure to complete schoolwork, and increased sleep). Although these avoidance behaviors help him manage in the moment, they further reinforce his depressive symptoms, and also result in a number of negative consequences, such as friends losing interest in spending time with him, and Peter's parents and teachers hassling him about his poor schoolwork. These negative consequences not only serve to reinforce the notion that Peter's "life circumstances" are less than desirable and rewarding, but they also feed into the vicious cycle of depressive symptoms, avoidance behaviors, and negative consequences, by adding to his negative life events and stressors.

Vignette 2

Zach is a smart 17-year-old boy who lives with his father, aunt, and uncle. Zach's parents divorced when he was 6, and Zach's mother lives with her longtime boyfriend, a man with whom she has two children. Zach cannot recall a time, since the age of 10, when he has not felt depressed, and to this end, endorses every symptom of MDD, including persistent sadness and irritability, anhedonia, appetite and sleep dysregulation, psychomotor retardation, worthlessness and guilt, poor concentration, and fatigue and loss of energy. Zach has struggled with suicidality for the last several years, and although he has never made a suicide attempt, he talks openly about ending his life using a range of different methods, including electrocuting himself. Although Zach lives in the same city as his mother, their visits are infrequent. Zach cherishes time with his mother but often feels disappointed by their visits, and notes that he feels like an "outsider" with her boyfriend and his half-siblings. In discussing Zach's situation with him, the therapist feels that his depression appears to be a large part of his identity, and he does not appear to be motivated to give up his depressive behavioral patterns. Zach's ongoing struggles with depression have not only alienated many of his peers but also, to some extent, his mother. He has few friends, and spends the large majority of his free time lamenting his mother's lack of involvement in his life, and looking at anime magazines and films, which he then criticizes for their "lack of originality and creativity." To this end, he frequently fantasizes about two things: (1) his parents getting back together and (2) the anime film he one day hopes to develop himself, complete with original art and story line.

Zach's Assessment Data

Zach provides an excellent example of a situation in which both parents and the youth not only agree that there is a problem, but also agree on the nature of the problem. Upon intake, both Zach and his father gave consistent reports with regard to Zach's presentation. Zach met criteria for major depression, and questionnaire data from both Zach and his father revealed scores within the clinically significant range on the SMFQ (total score = 23) and SMFQ–Parent (total score = 17), and on the Anxious–Depressed scale of the YSR (*T*-score = 73) and CBCL (*T*-score = 70). Zach's difficulties with suicidality were reflected in his score of 80 on the SIQ, placing him at the 97th percentile, with Zach's father emphasizing his worry about Zach's potential for making a suicide attempt. Neither Zach nor his father noted any concerns with regard to externalizing behaviors on the YSR (*T*-score = 45) and CBCL (*T*-score = 43).

Zach's Case Conceptualization

The "life circumstances" contributing to Zach's long-standing sense of depression (see Figure 2.4) seem to be tied to his sense of having lost his connection with his mother at the age of 6, when his parents divorced. Since that time, he has seen her infrequently and when he does, he tends to feel like an "outsider" with her and her new family. This has ultimately led Zach to experience his severe depressive symptoms (see "How do you feel?" in Figure 2.4), including symptoms such as sadness, irritability, anhedonia,

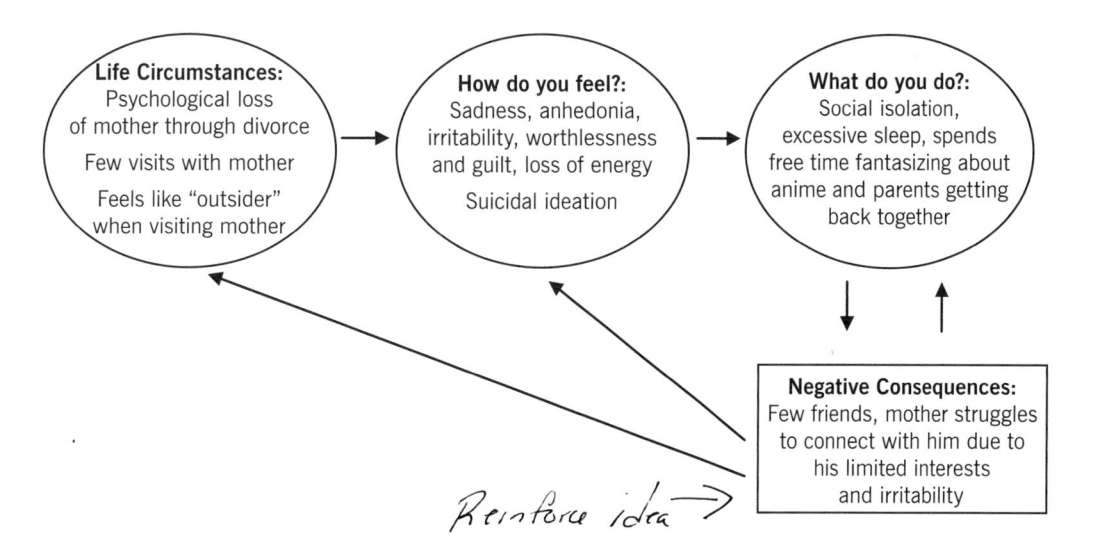

FIGURE 2.4. Zach's case conceptualization within the BA model.

and feelings of worthlessness and excessive guilt, poor concentration, and loss of energy. Zach's response to his depressive feelings (see "What do you do?" in Figure 2.4) has been to retreat into himself, isolate himself from those around him, sleep whenever possible, and find refuge in fantasy. While these avoidance behaviors serve to help him manage in the moment, they only reinforce Zach's depressive symptoms and further result in a number of negative consequences (see "Negative Consequences" box in Figure 2.4), in that he has alienated himself from peers and his mother with his ongoing and severe depressive symptoms and limited interests outside of anime. These negative consequences serve both to reinforce the notion that his life circumstances are unrewarding and further feed into the cycle of depressive symptoms, avoidance behaviors, and negative consequences by adding to Zach's negative life circumstances.

Vignette 3

Eva is a 17-year-old girl who lives with her biological parents. She also has an adult sister who lives locally with her husband, and with whom Eva is close. Eva has always been shy, but as a young child, she typically had some friends both at school and in her neighborhood. She was frequently invited to birthday parties and other group events but rarely was invited for one-on-one sleepovers and did not initiate inviting others over to her house despite her parents' encouragement to do so. The academic and social aspects of high school initially challenged her. Eva largely adjusts to academic demands, typically earning average to above-average grades, but she has never developed very strong friendships. Throughout her childhood, Eva's parents enrolled her in sports and dance classes; however, by high school, these activities have fallen by the wayside as extracurricular activities became more competitive and selective. Eva participates in a church youth group but otherwise reports frequent boredom and difficulty finding ways to keep herself busy. She reports spending most of her free time online watching YouTube videos and television shows. She denies any history of romantic relationships or interest in having a romantic relationship. In the context of working on her senior project, a volunteer project followed by a class presentation about the experience, Eva has begun to report somatic symptoms of anxiety and frequent headaches and stomachaches, resulting in many days of missed school. When her mother confronts her about whether she is trying to avoid school, Eva discloses that in fact she is struggling with schoolwork generally and has a lot of fear about her senior project, including the steps required to set up her volunteer work, conducting the work and, most of all, presenting it at the end of the year. Upon seeking mental health services, Eva further reports feeling socially isolated and sad. She also endorses experiencing poor concentration, initial insomnia, fatigue, irritability, low self-esteem, crying spells, and some vague and passive thoughts of death.

Eva's Assessment Data

Eva's case provides an example in which an adolescent endorses problems and difficulties about which her parents are not aware, likely due to the fact that she is focused on her internal experiences and her parents have focused more on what they observe.

Upon clinical interview and the completion of a range of questionnaires, Eva's therapist diagnosed her with an unspecified depressive disorder and an unspecified anxiety disorder. The diagnoses, however, were largely determined by Eva's report and not that of her mother. For example, while Eva's clinical interview responses were highly suggestive of a depressive disorder, her mother's report did not necessarily indicate that this was the case. Likewise, this was the pattern seen on various self-report measures, with Eva's SMFQ (total score = 11) indicating difficulties with depressive symptoms while her mother's responses did not (SMFQ–Parent total score = 3). Similarly, indices of anxiety symptoms indicated difficulties via Eva's report (YSR Anxious–Depressed T-score = 72) and fewer concerns via parental report (CBCL Anxious–Depressed T-Score = 60). The only thing that Eva and her mother agreed on was a low risk of suicide (SIQ total score = 4, 29th percentile), despite Eva's self-reported vague thoughts of death (e.g., wondering who might attend whose funeral if an adolescent at her school died). Behavioral observations made during the assessment led the therapist to feel comfortable in relying more heavily on Eva's report. Eva presented as a shy, anxious adolescent who appeared significantly sad, and who could adequately report on her own internal experience, whereas Eva's mother reported that she struggled to understand what was going on with Eva, because her daughter did not share much and she [the mother] could only rely on what she could see (e.g., missing school with complaints of headaches and stomachaches).

Eva's Case Conceptualization

The A-BAP case conceptualization for Eva is summarized in Figure 2.5. The life circumstances contributing to Eva's difficulties center around long-standing social anxiety that has resulted in a lack of close friendships and school pressures related to managing the significant academic demands of high school. These issues/concerns have ultimately led Eva to feel sad and irritable, with accompanying fatigue and thoughts of self-harm and suicide (see "What do you feel?" in Figure 2.5), and in response to these feelings, she has

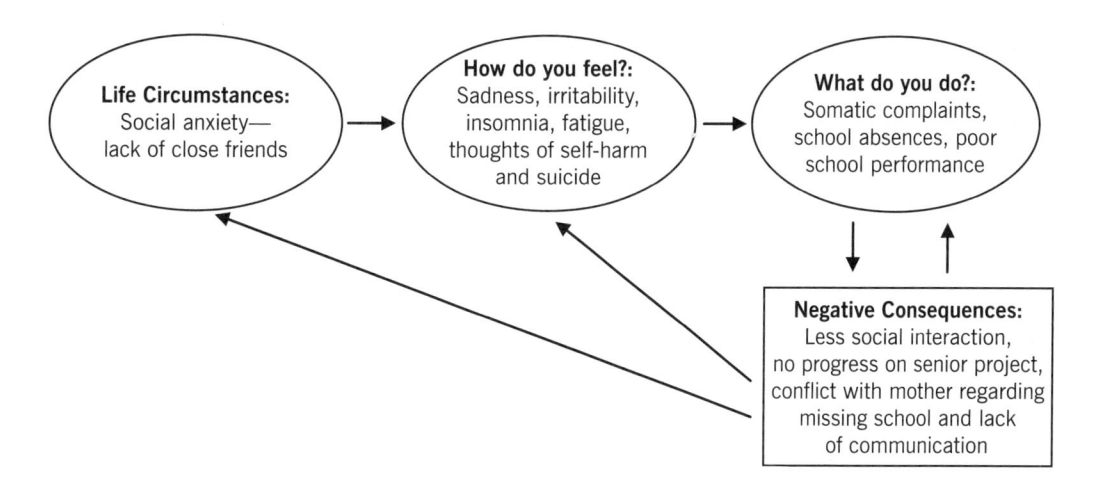

FIGURE 2.5. Eva's case conceptualization within the BA model.

had a tendency to retreat into numerous somatic complaints without physical foundation that have in turn resulted in school absences and declining grades (see "What do you do?" in Figure 2.5). As with the cases of both Peter and Zach, Eva's response to her feelings of depression have resulted in a number of "negative consequences," including little social interaction, lack of progress on her senior project, and conflict with her mother regarding school absences. This, in turn, has created a negative feedback loop, not only reinforcing her view of her life as one that has few rewards but also further reinforcing her ever-increasing feelings of depression and thoughts of self-harm and suicide.

Vignette 4

Rebecca is a 15-year-old girl who lives with her mother. She spends time with her father every other weekend and typically sees him a few days during the week, because he helps coach her soccer team and provides transportation to all soccer-related activities. Rebecca has two siblings—a 10-year-old sister who lives with Rebecca and her mother and a 17-year-old brother who lives with her father. Rebecca's growth and development has been problem-free, although she began showing signs of puberty a bit earlier than her peers and was fully developed, having started her menstrual cycle, by the end of sixth grade. During elementary and early middle school, Rebecca was a solid student, and her parents described her as "sunny and outgoing," with lots of friends and activities. Her parents further reported that she "changed dramatically" during seventh grade, and Rebecca herself admits that she began to feel more left out by friends and less motivated to keep up with her schoolwork at that time. When her closest friend moved away at the beginning of eighth grade, Rebecca began hanging out with kids whom her parents describe as "troublemakers." Although she kept up with soccer, Rebecca's grades started dropping, she became increasingly irritable, especially when asked to participate in family activities with either parent, and spent all her time on the Internet or texting friends. Rebecca began to skip school on occasion, got caught drinking on a few occasions, and snuck out of the house to "hang out" with a boy her parents felt was too old and "streetwise" for her. She is now in her first year of high school, and although initially excited about the transition, Rebecca reports feeling overwhelmed with her schoolwork, the social demands, and "all the drama." She has had more and more trouble getting to sleep at night, and as a result, often struggles to get up for school the next morning and reports feeling tired all the time. Rebecca's mother is not only worried about her schoolwork but she also worries about Rebecca's negative attitude and withdrawal from activities—even getting her to go to soccer has been a struggle. Right before winter break, the boy she liked started to hang out with a female friend, and Rebecca reported feeling ugly and hopeless. Rebecca snuck a bottle of aspirin into her room one night with thoughts of suicide but got scared and told her mother about how bad she was feeling.

Rebecca's Assessment Data

Rebecca's case highlights the importance of therapists sorting through co-occurring symptoms, as well as deciphering whether some symptoms are representative of transient developmental phenomena or of clinical concern in their own right. Rebecca clearly qualifies for a diagnosis of MDD based on both her own and her parents responses during a clinical interview, as well as reports on the SMFQ (total score = 17 and SMFQ–Parent total score = 15). Rebecca, however, also displays some co-occurring externalizing symptoms (e.g., sneaking out of the house, getting caught drinking) that need to be considered in understanding her treatment needs. While reports of externalizing symptoms by Rebecca on the YSR (T-score = 63) were not too concerning, reports of her parents (CBCL T-score = 70) were clinically significant. In addition, a screen of Rebecca's drug and alcohol use suggested the need for further evaluation. After interviewing both Rebecca and her parents in depth with regard to these issues, it was determined that Rebecca did not meet the criteria for any type of disruptive behavior or substance abuse/dependence disorder, and these symptoms were likely more a function of adolescent experimentation and her underlying depression. The therapist, however, made note of them, with a plan to check-in about them frequently and, if appropriate, make them treatment targets as Rebecca participated in the A-BAP.

Rebecca's Case Conceptualization

The A-BAP case conceptualization for Rebecca is depicted in Figure 2.6. Specifically, Rebecca's case highlights the "buildup" of stress over time. Her exposure to multiple stressors may have had a cumulative effect on Rebecca and overtaxed her coping abilities. While Rebecca's loss of her friends in the eighth grade seemed important to the start of her downward spiral, most recently, her life circumstances and stressors have involved peer pressure, academic stress with the transition to high school, and rejection by a boy. These circumstances and stressors have led to feelings of irritability, anhedonia, fatigue, worthlessness, and suicidal ideation (see "How do you feel?" in Figure 2.6) and resulted in Rebecca withdrawing from family and friends, skipping school and sports activities, and escaping through substance use (see "What do you do?" in Figure 2.6). Rebecca's responses to her feelings of depression have resulted in a number of "negative

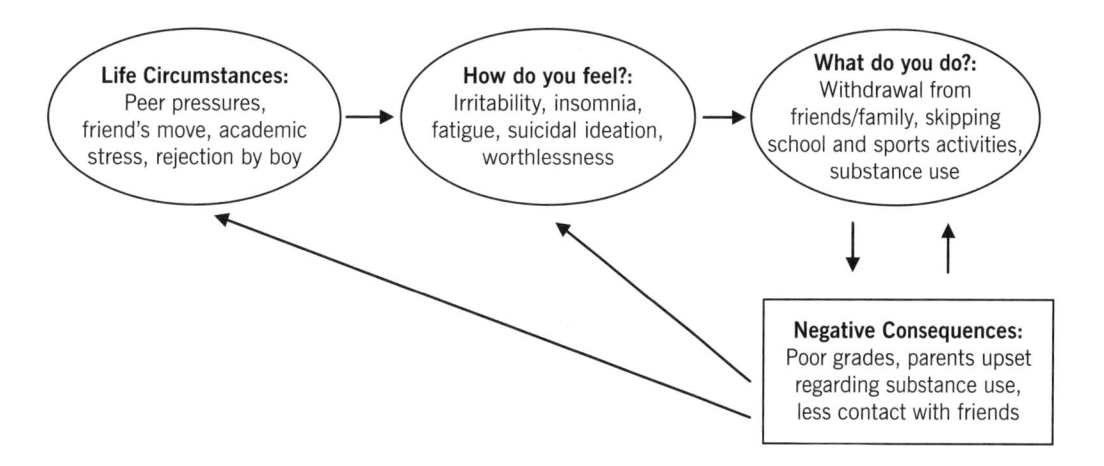

FIGURE 2.6. Rebecca's case conceptualization within the BA model.

consequences" with poor grades, her parents upset regarding her substance use, and loss of contact with peers.

Treatment Planning

Treatment planning is always driven by case conceptualization. In the cases outlined here, the unique aspects of each case conceptualization are coupled with the hypothesized mechanism of change in the model to formulate a treatment plan. The hypothesized mechanism of change in the BA model centers on response-contingent positive reinforcement (RCPR). More specifically, the BA model of change highlights that (1) as barriers to activation are identified and addressed, the adolescent's ability to engage fully in activities and experience RCPR will be enhanced; (2) repeated trials of activation will increase the likelihood that these activities will be experienced as positively reinforcing even in the face of initial negative mood; and (3) when activities are positively reinforcing, it is anticipated that depressive symptoms will abate (McCauley, Schloredt, Gudmundsen, Martell, and Dimidjian, 2015). With this in mind, treatment planning is collaboratively designed with the adolescent and starts with a thorough review of the BA model and how the "life circumstances" and subsequent experiences of each adolescent fit into that model (as outlined earlier). Starting with a discussion about what has been happening and the "life circumstances" of each youth, the therapist then moved on to discuss how those "life circumstances" impacted the mood of each adolescent and how those feelings were connected with what he or she did, and to examine how those feelings and actions often led to negative consequences and ultimately kept the youth stuck in the vicious cycle of depression. While to some therapists this may feel like a rote application of the model, there are always unique aspects to each case that require great care and attention from the therapist as he or she develops the treatment plan to engage the adolescent in skill building. For example, with Peter, it would be strongly recommended that the therapist discuss Peter's depression with him without labeling his feelings and behaviors as "depression," because Peter did not describe himself in those terms, and focus instead on a more concrete aspect of his difficulties that Peter might be willing to acknowledge and work on, such as his parent's concern about dropping grades; this will likely help Peter buy into the model and engage him more from the start, even though the techniques utilized will not differ. For Zach, Eva, and Rebecca, on the other hand, the therapist could talk more openly about depression and what it means to each of these youth, because they had little difficulty with the notion of labeling their struggles as "depression."

After a thorough review of the case conceptualization in the context of the BA model, the therapist for each adolescent would then begin to utilize a series of didactic experiences to help each adolescent understand his or her situation more thoroughly and in real time. In the A-BAP, the starting point always centers on activation. Key to the focus on activation is helping the adolescent understand that the natural human response to feelings of depression are, in fact, avoidance behaviors—increased sleep, anergia, isolation, lack of motivation around task demand—that feel good, as if they are the solution to depressive feelings. These ultimately end up reinforcing a worsening of symptoms, either directly by virtue of their impact on depressive feelings (e.g., when the adolescent sleeps outside of normal sleeping hours, she or he often wakes up feeling tired; when the adolescent isolates and feels more lonely) or indirectly through negative consequences (e.g., when the adolescent isolates, friends quit calling, leading to more sad and lonely feelings; when the adolescent is not motivated to engage in schoolwork, and parents and teachers get upset, the youth feels more pressure, and as if he or she is letting others down). Ultimately, it involves working with the adolescent to identify another behavioral response (one that may result in RCPR) in the face of depressive feelings—something he or she is willing to try that could also be more rewarding and encouraging to him or her. Given Peter's propensity to isolate himself and not complete his schoolwork, this might mean working with him to take one small step, such as homework for one class for one week, which in turn might expose him to positive feedback and help him begin to recognize that he can, in fact, feel better, even if only momentarily, by being more engaged and working toward goals. This might mean helping Zach connect his depressive symptoms to the loss of quality time with his mother and come to his own conclusion that his isolation, excessive sleep, and retreat into fantasy only serve to alienate him from the people, like his mother, with whom he desperately wants to engage. With this, the therapist would need to work diligently to help Zach identify some alternative behaviors he would be willing to try or "experiment with" to see if he can feel better, even if only for a fleeting moment. Over the course of treatment, the therapist might work with Zach to develop a realistic and gradual plan (i.e., generate mini-steps) to establish consistent quality time with his mother.

In helping each adolescent draw connections among situations, activities, and moods and realize the important difference between mood- and goal-directed behavior, the therapist will ask him or her to track activity, as well as mood, and based on patterns observed, begin to plan some activities as a way to combat times in which he or she may be particularly vulnerable to engaging in avoidance behaviors, again with the goal of engaging in repeated trials of activation. For example, given Eva's social anxiety and lack of close relationships that add to her feelings of depression, she would, for starters, be asked to track what is going on around her (situations), how she feels (mood), and what she does (activity). She and her therapist would then look for patterns of behavior and discuss alternative activities that she might be willing to try, with the notion of observing the impact on her mood. This may start with some simple experiments that center around sending some text messages to peers to initially show interest (e.g., "Can you believe all the homework we got in Algebra today?"), then, over time, increase the complexity of those messages (e.g., "Would you be interested in studying for our Algebra test together after school?"). This would then lead to the use of other techniques related to helping her set some specific goals, such as asking a peer at school to engage in a social activity unrelated to school, and identifying the mini-steps she might take to work up to that goal.

The therapist will undoubtedly be required to discuss concepts in terms that each individual adolescent can relate to and embrace. For example, Peter not only minimized his depressive symptoms but also often pooh-poohed a number of concepts. More specifically, Peter struggled with the concept of goal setting, arguing that goals required no special planning and that mini-steps were not needed to achieve a goal. After a few sessions in which Peter could not embrace the concept of goal setting, the therapist, knowing Peter's interest in football, applied the concept of goal setting to how a football play would get called in a game (e.g., the quarterback gets the call from the sideline and communicates the play to his team, all the players line up, the quarterback calls the play, the team executes the play). This unique application turned the tide for Peter and not only could he understand the concept of goal setting and mini-steps, but following this, Peter and his therapist framed all of his goals in the context of a play. While the overarching goals of the A-BAP are consistent for all youth, the manner in which the therapist gets there is flexible. Ultimately the treatment plan is meant to guide the therapist to an end goal (to decrease depression through RCPR). It is not meant to be applied so rigidly that it ignores the unique needs of the adolescent in the process. That is, if an adolescent needs more time with a particular concept, more time should be allowed. The onus that is on the therapist, however, is to work continually to apply BA principles to everything that the adolescent brings forward in treatment. For example, if the therapist was planning to focus on goal setting, but Rebecca reported that she was not going to the school football game with her friends for fear that she might see the boy who rejected her, the therapist might choose to steer the discussion to focus on goal- versus mood-directed behavior (a topic that may have been introduced in an earlier session), then apply the concept of goal setting to Rebecca's specific situation. This is a task that seems less and less formidable the more the therapist utilizes the concepts and has experience with the model.

Summary

Assessment, case conceptualization, and treatment planning are the cornerstones of any intervention program, and the same is true for the A-BAP. Assessment of youth should follow an MTMM approach, whenever possible. Such assessment not only informs decision making with regard to diagnosis and the appropriateness of youth for the A-BAP, but it also further feeds directly into the A-BAP case conceptualization. This case conceptualization, in turn, informs treatment planning and the individualized application of the BA model to the unique needs and clinical presentation of the adolescent. Although A-BAP is not an appropriate treatment for all youth, depressed youth, with and without mild suicidality and some co-occurring symptoms, are excellent candidates for the program.

CHAPTER 3

How to Use the A-BAP Session Guides

As we stressed in Chapter 2, in working within the BA model, the therapist's first charge is to develop an idiographic case conceptualization that leads to an individualized application of the BA model to the unique circumstances of each adolescent. As new information and a more nuanced understanding of the adolescent's perspective unfolds over time, the individual case conceptualization and individualized BA treatment plan shift to accommodate new input. This chapter focuses on the practical aspects of using the BA approach with adolescents and determining how best to individualize treatment to the needs of each adolescent. The chapter explains the "how to" of using the material outlined in each module and session, with examples of the ways in which each treatment element can be tailored to fit the needs of adolescents encountered in clinical practice. We close with a discussion of key BA elements that can be integrated within the context of clinical care that does not specifically use the A-BAP program.

As outlined in this volume, in each of the first eight sessions, key concepts and related skills are introduced. The concepts are generally straightforward, not difficult to understand, and take little time to communicate. The challenge is both to help the adolescent see how these concepts could be useful in day-to-day struggles and to motivate him or her to apply the concepts (and related skills) to cope with challenging life situations. To accomplish this, it is essential that the therapist work to become facile at drawing examples that are pertinent to each adolescent into the presentation of the concepts, skills, and out-of-session practice activity specified in each week's "Test It Out" activity. It always is more effective to communicate an idea or skill while working through an example from the adolescent's own experience, although it may be best to start with examples that are not too personal, anxiety provoking, or distressing. Over time, the therapist can encourage the adolescent to apply skills to more central and significant problem areas.

Although the skills are included in a specific order within modules and sessions, it may be helpful to modify this order to fit the needs of the adolescent. Highly reactive adolescents may benefit from an early introduction of the COPE (Calm and Clarify, Options, Perform, Evaluate) approach to problem solving, with special attention to emotion regulation techniques. In some cases, the therapist may also want to bring in other evidence-based strategies to address specific problems with which the adolescent is coping, such as more intensive exposure or habit reversal training. It is fine to do this if the therapist provides a clear rationale and has the time and skill to carry out the needed added intervention component effectively. Many of these issues, such as social avoidance/anxiety, can be readily addressed in the context of barriers that get in the way of moving toward valued goals.

The session guides also include handouts that illustrate key concepts or help structure the "Test It Out" activity. Some adolescents like referring to handouts, whereas others do not. The handouts can be found on pages 173–211, and we encourage the therapist to review them before each session and individualize their use to the needs/preferences of the individual adolescent. In our experience, use of at least some selected forms works best. The handouts are there to support and guide, not to dictate how the therapist does the work. In our experience, adolescents do engage in the out-of-session exercises included in this protocol; however, engagement only occurs if the therapist troubleshoots barriers to completing the "Test It Out" activity when it is presented and reviews the activity in the next session (even if the adolescent did not complete the assignment. Many sessions also include some time to check-in or teach a skill to the parent. It is fine to manage this work in a way that best fits the needs of the adolescent and parent, the context of therapy, and the therapist's style—parent material can be presented in conjoint sessions with the adolescent, held for a subsequent session in the face of time constraints, covered in separately scheduled meetings with parents, or reviewed in a phone consultation if working in a context (e.g., school) where parents may not be readily available.

Module 1: Getting Started (Sessions 1 and 2)

This module includes two sessions designed to educate the adolescent and parent about the overall structure and assumptions of therapy within the BA approach.

Session 1: Introduction to the Adolescent Behavioral Activation Program (A-BAP)

The therapy typically begins with the adolescent and his or her parent/guardian together, but this can be varied based on the context of treatment and the needs and preferences of the therapist, adolescent, and/or family. The therapist outlines concrete issues, including confidentiality, frequency and spacing of treatment sessions, length of sessions, structure of sessions (i.e., that they include time with the adolescent, time with parents to either check-in, or time to work with the parent and adolescent together). The therapist also outlines adolescent, therapist, and parent roles in BA in order to establish clearly that the adolescent is the active agent of change in his or her life, and the therapist and parent are both there to encourage, guide, and support the adolescent in the change process.

The therapist's role is not to tell the adolescent what to do or simply listen to his or her concerns but instead to teach strategies that might be useful, then "coach" the adolescent as therapist and adolescent collaboratively fine-tune strategies to fit the adolescent's situation and/or style. Parents are encouraged to provide instrumental support by helping adolescents (especially younger adolescents) access activities, events, and resources they have identified as ways to get more socially or academically engaged, and to provide emotional support for adolescents' efforts to try new solutions or behaviors. It is also important to plant the seed that BA is an active treatment modality that calls on the adolescent (and sometimes the parent) to experiment with new approaches or strategies outside of therapy. This is reflected in the "Test It Out" activities or experiments that are part of each session and serve as an essential way of learning what might work to alleviate the adolescent's distress. Within the BA model, this material is presented in a friendly, collegial manner meant to normalize the experiences of the adolescent and demystify therapy. This tone can be communicated via comments such as "Everyone struggles with feeling down sometimes" or "We will work together to learn some strategies that might be helpful, just like you might work with a coach to get better at soccer."

Next, the therapist introduces the BA model. The therapist may use the Handout 1 "Behavioral Activation Model" teaching guide or walk through each component in a more casual fashion. We have found that a visual depiction of the model, either with the handout or simply drawing it on paper or a whiteboard, helps to maximize clear communication and understanding. Once the overall model is presented, it is also useful to walk through the Handout 2 worksheet "How Behavioral Activation Works for You," encouraging the adolescent and his or her parent to suggest examples that are pertinent to the individual adolescent, but not pushing for a level of disclosure with which the adolescent is not comfortable. At this point in therapy, we assume that the adolescent, parent, and therapist will be drawing on information from an initial intake or evaluation process. Thus, it is important to respect what the adolescent or parent might or might not be comfortable sharing in the conjoint session format. This session is designed to engage the adolescent and family in part by carefully listening to their "story" and outlining how the BA approach will address their needs. The goal is to give them a sense of the model that will guide the work of therapy, not to engage in an in-depth discussion of family stressors, parent–adolescent conflicts, or the adolescent's shortcomings. If the interaction between parent and adolescent is strained, it can be best to just walk through the model using an "example" adolescent, with the therapist taking the lead and filling in the material.

In the last part of this session, the therapist meets alone with the adolescent to introduce some additional components that will characterize their work together. First, the therapist explains the use of a brief symptom checklist for the adolescent to complete at the beginning of each session, which helps identify difficulties to work on in treatment and keep track of the extent to which the adolescent's symptoms are changing over time. Second, the therapist introduces the idea of an agenda to determine how to allocate time in each session. It is important to encourage the adolescent to use the agenda-setting time to identify issues on which he or she wants to focus. It also is important for the therapist to honor the adolescent's potential need to talk about his or her thoughts and feelings, while also moving forward to learn and practice change strategies; agenda setting helps to balance such considerations. Finally, the therapist introduces the "Test It Out" activities that will be part of every session. The goal is to begin with simple tasks that do not feel too burdensome to the adolescent but that begin his or her engagement in attending to things outside of sessions that affect his or her mood. For each "Test It Out" activity, we have included a form or worksheet for the adolescent (and sometimes the parents) to use. These can be used if they make sense in the treatment context or fit with the adolescent's style. If not, it is fine to create individualized ways of tracking the information, such as using the adolescent's phone. It is critical to anticipate barriers to completing the out-of-session activities and to make sure the tasks are shaped to fit the adolescent's needs and preferences. The "Test It Out" activity (Handout 3: "Activity Monitoring") suggested in the first session tracks how the adolescent is spending his or her time. It is helpful for the therapist to orient to this task in a nonjudgmental fashion, explaining the rationale that paying attention to what he or she is doing can help to clarify how feelings and mood are affected by what the adolescent does. The task is started in the session, so that the therapist can guide the adolescent, answer questions, and make sure that the task seems easy to do and not too invasive or taxing.

Session 2: Situation–Activity–Mood Cycle

The second "Getting Started" session is spent primarily with the adolescent, although a brief check-in with parents is included at the end. The goal of the session is to gain an understanding of the adolescent's current relationships and activities and to help the adolescent identify and understand the connection between activities and mood—that what we do affects how we feel. As with all subsequent sessions, the second session begins with a brief check-in that includes completion and review of the self-report mood questionnaire and the development of an agenda for the session. To set the agenda, the therapist can elicit issues the adolescent wants to talk about, outline information the therapist wants to cover, and allot time as needed. The session introduces two key concepts. The first is how relationships and activities affect mood and begins with an assessment of what people and activities are important to the adolescent, using, if helpful, the Handout 4 worksheet "Who and What Is on 'First' in Your Life?". This assessment draws on an approach used in IPT-A (Mufson et al., 2004) and is designed to ensure that the therapist has a good understanding of the adolescent's social context given the importance of social interactions during adolescence (Slavich, 2014). The second concept focuses on understanding that the ways in which we respond to difficult situations can trigger either a downward or an upward mood spiral.

Even if the adolescent presents with a pressing problem to discuss, it is important not to abandon review of the "Test It Out" task from the previous session, introduction of new material/skills, or the "Test It Out" work for the week to come. The review of both the "Test It Out" task and the new skills can be brief, if need be, and the new "Test It Out" assignment can be tailored to reflect an issue the adolescent has raised. For example, Rebecca (as presented in Chapter 2) states at the beginning of Session 2 that she wants to talk about running into her "new" friends at the mall that weekend and feeling left out, more depressed, and worthless. It will be important to allow time to talk this through, but it is equally important, and very timely, to integrate this information into her discussion of who is important in her life and how they help or hinder her mood. The therapist might ask if her weekend's experience changes how she sees these friends and their ability to influence her mood. The difficulty of Rebecca's real-life situation should not only be validated but also should be presented as an opportunity for new learning, since she and her therapist can use it to walk through the situation (seeing peers), her reaction and what she did, and how she felt and collaboratively come up with some actions that Rebecca could try to lighten her mood again. Her example can be acknowledged in planning the "Test It Out" activity (Handout 5: "Downward Spiral, Upward Spiral") for the week to come by incorporating some positive things she could do to take care of herself should she run into another peer problem that triggers a downward spiral.

The session with the adolescent ends with a transition to a brief meeting with parents to provide some psychoeducation about adolescent depression by giving them the Handout 6 teaching guide "A Parent Guide to Adolescent Depression." The goal is to provide support for the parents, as well as to place the adolescent's challenging behaviors (withdrawal, irritability) in the context of depression. It is helpful to emphasize that such behaviors are not willful or rejecting, and that they are not behaviors that the adolescent can simply "turn on or off." The time with parents ends with a brief review of ways to support the adolescent. For example, in the case of Rebecca, with Rebecca's permission, time with parents could include identifying ways they might support her if peer rejection pops up again. The goal is to acknowledge that when adolescents are depressed, their parents often are perplexed by their behavior and vulnerable to misinterpretation, including sometimes even taking adolescents' irritability and withdrawal as a personal attack against them and the family. Reframing such behavior and helping the parents understand it as "the depression talking" can go a long way in mobilizing parents' abilities to support the adolescent through this difficult time.

Module 2: Getting Active (Sessions 3 and 4)

The two sessions in this module introduce the role of BA in mood management, with attention to understanding the short- and long-term consequences of behavioral choices.

Session 3: Goal-Directed versus Mood-Directed Behavior

This session continues the activity–mood focus of Session 2, underscoring that activity can be used to change mood *and* that some activities make us feel better, while others make us feel worse. The first key concept introduced is the idea of mood-directed versus goal-directed behavior and the importance of getting active even when one's mood is down. After walking through the Handout 7 teaching guide "Getting Active!," we have suggested an in-session exercise to clarify the key points. This involves engaging the adolescent in a brief "experiment" to see whether he or she notices even a tiny change in mood after watching a funny or touching YouTube video, listening to an upbeat song, taking a brisk walk, and so forth. This should be introduced as an experiment with a "let's see" attitude and the acknowledgment that it may or may not "work." The therapist can engage the adolescent in identifying the activity that might shift mood. Such a conversation (e.g., identifying the types of humorous YouTube clips the adolescent has enjoyed) itself can shift mood. If this occurs, highlighting the shift in mood can help demonstrate how simple activities can have an impact. It is important for the therapist to participate actively in this experiment, rating his or her own mood and modeling honestly any changes noted. Some adolescents easily engage in this exercise, while others are self-conscious or too shut down to want to try almost anything. Simple things like listening to a song or eating a piece of candy may be small steps in the attempt to make the point if an adolescent is emotionally shut down or reluctant to try new things. The therapist should always be mindful of, accept, and label a "no change" response as useful information.

The second concept is simply extending the activity monitoring introduced in Session 1 to activity–mood monitoring as a way to learn what activities help to shift the adolescent's mood in a more positive or negative direction. The difference with this "Test It Out" exercise is that the adolescent is asked to track feelings, as well as activities. As with activity monitoring, we suggest that the therapist begin this as an in-session activity, so that he or she can help adolescents identify times when they notice even a small shift in mood related to a change in what they were doing (e.g., talking with a friend at lunch vs. sitting alone at assembly). This leads into introducing the "Test It Out" activity, using the Handout 8 worksheet "Activity–Mood Chart—Example" and Handout 9 "Activity–Mood Chart" to structure the "Test-It-Out" task choosing a few days in the week to track activities and mood.

This session also includes a parent education component using the Handout 10 worksheet "Ways to Describe Parenting an Adolescent." It is important for the therapist to let the adolescent know what he or she will be talking about with the adolescent's parent, and that he or she will not be bringing up the adolescent's personal issues or concerns. If the adolescent has something for the therapist to discuss with the parents, then it is always good to try to do that in a session that includes the adolescent in order to model open communication and problem solving. As in Session 2, time constraints may mean that the parent component is done at a different time; over the phone; or, again, within the context of a meeting that includes the adolescent.

Session 4: Introducing Consequences of Behavior

Session 4 introduces functional analysis in a way that is easy to understand using the frame of "why I do what I do" and continues laying the groundwork for effective activity scheduling. The session begins, as always, with completion and review of a symptom checklist, the agenda, and the "Test It Out" activity from the last session. The adolescent's individual issues should be woven into each of these activities and into the discussion of the session's new concepts. Session 4 includes more material than prior sessions (four rather than two key concepts) and may need to be broken down into smaller components if the adolescent adds to the agenda, if the therapist has limited time with the adolescent, or if the adolescent does better when less information is presented and more time is allocated to talk through things. In this case, the therapist would cover the material over several sessions rather than trying to accomplish everything in one. We have found that it is typically feasible to introduce all of the concepts, barring any big issues the adolescent may need to add to the agenda.

The first key concept introduces analyses of the payoff versus price of a behavior, which builds on understanding "why I do what I do." In the case of Peter in Chapter 2, this discussion might underscore the "payoff" and "price" of how he has coped with his brother. For instance, even though it makes sense for Peter to avoid upsetting his brother given the high "price" of putting up with his tantrums, it might be useful for Peter also to evaluate the "payoff" versus the "price" of avoiding time with friends.

The next section extends the discussion of payoff versus price to include consideration of the short- versus long-term consequences of behavior using the Handout 11 teaching guide "Short- versus Long-Term Consequences." Attention is given here to the idea that behaviors that might improve mood in the short term can sometimes have a longer-term price (e.g., avoiding homework by going online feels good in the moment but perhaps not the next day in class). Other behaviors may be hard in the short term (e.g., the high price of studying for a test) but pay off in the long term (e.g., getting a good grade). The third concept introduces the idea of using activities to control your mood, beginning with a more in-depth focus on the core BA skill of activity scheduling. In BA, activity scheduling goes beyond simply adding in more "pleasant events." Using the Handout 12 worksheet "Pump You Up, Bring You Down," the essential work is to collaborate with the adolescent to identify activities that are tied to his or her personal goals and values—that is, activities that are rewarding for him or her. Although the concepts of goals and values may be complicated for some younger adolescents, the therapist can keep it simple by helping the adolescent to articulate what he or she wants and what is important to him or her. Although initial discussions may focus on everyday activities, it is important to work to engage the adolescent in a thoughtful assessment of what kinds of things he or she uniquely values and likes to do—stepping-stones to these activities are what the therapist wants the adolescent, over time, to build back into his or her life. This process begins in this session with a consideration of what kinds of activities are associated with positive ("pump you up") versus negative ("bring you down") mood, and an initial discussion of the wide variety of activities one can engage in to combat a negative mood. The Handout 13 teaching guide "Activities Menu" can be used to help generate ideas.

To conclude the session's focus on functional analysis of behavior, we include a brief practice exercise to concretize the importance of attending to and enjoying positive activities, even if momentary, as a way to bolster mood when feeling down or in the midst of a negative situation. This is also meant to activate the adolescent in session and move away from being too didactic. As noted earlier, this is a full session, so the timing will have to be adapted to the adolescent's needs and the therapist's style. The presentation of this idea of "making the most of a good feeling" is best if it can be worked into a brief "experiment" in the session. When talking about activities that appeal to adolescents, simply ask them to do a quick rating of their current mood, then to think about a time when they were happily engaged in one of their named activities—ask them to describe who they were with; the sounds, smells, colors, and feelings; and what made it enjoyable. Help them bask in the "good" feeling for a just few minutes, then do another mood rating.

In rating "mood," the therapist can select whatever term is most effective with each adolescent. For example, considering Peter's case again, since he might not be able/willing to rate depression per se, the therapist might use a term that makes the most sense for him (e.g., *energy, irritability,* or *interest*) and ask him to rate it before and after describing a time when he was actively engaged in one of the "pump you up" activities he listed, perhaps something fun with friends. In the context of this "experiment" in session, the therapist can help the adolescent draw out the details, share the pleasant memory, and talk about the importance of attending to positive times and memories, which can sometimes foster a positive mood.

We end this session with a "Test It Out" assignment, using Handout 14 "Activities That Help to PUMP You Up!!" to schedule in one or two "pump you up activities." While this task may seem simple, it is the first activity scheduling assignment and must therefore be set up with some care. To this end, it is important to allow enough time to walk through the following steps:

- Work collaboratively with the adolescent to identify what activity or activities to schedule. This may be readily apparent from discussion during the session or it may need a bit more time to flesh out—the goal is to find something that has meaning to the young person, so that he or she is not just "going through the motions" or choosing something he or she can easily "blow off."
- Talk through task difficulty and, if needed, break the activity down into smaller, doable parts. The goal is to try something that is a bit of a challenge but not overwhelming. It may take some discussion to get to the "sweet spot," but that discussion is important.
- Work with the adolescent to get at least one activity concretely scheduled. Specifically, walk the adolescent through the "who, what, where, when, and why" (the five W's) for each activity. This should be done in a lighthearted manner but with clear intent to help the adolescent "visualize" actually engaging in the activity.
- Identify and troubleshoot barriers to engaging in the activities.
- Set up a system to monitor the link between activities and mood.

These steps can all be done in a casual and conversational way that is not too time-consuming. As always, set it up as an experiment, with the goal of attending to what the adolescent learns from the process. The assignment also asks the adolescent to track a time when he or she felt good and practice "holding on to it" by texting a friend or taking a picture.

Module 3: Skill Building (Sessions 5–8)

In the third module, four key concepts and related skills (problem solving, goal setting, identifying barriers, and overcoming avoidance) are introduced. Again, all sessions in this module begin with the usual check-in, monitoring of symptoms, development of a shared agenda, and review of the "Test It Out" activity from the previous session.

Session 5: Problem Solving

The suggested structure for Session 5 involves spending about half the time with the adolescent, teaching a simple approach to problem solving, followed by an equal amount of time with the parents. The basic steps in problem solving are presented to the adolescent using the acronym COPE outlined in the Handout 15 teaching guide "Using COPE to Solve Problems." The "C" stands for "Calm and Clarify," and the therapist begins by talking with the adolescent about the importance of being calm before deciding on what actions to take when feeling upset or facing a problem. Common stress management techniques (counting, breathing, muscle relaxation, distraction) are reviewed and/or taught depending on the needs of each youth. In our experience, many adolescents have already been exposed to these strategies, which allows for a brief review and identification of the favored "go to" strategy. Once the asolescent is calm, the therapist and adolescent clarify the problem at hand, because first reactions may cloud understanding of the actual problem that needs to be solved. The next two steps involve generating and examining Options (the "O") in relation to payoff, price, short- and long-term consequences, and selecting and Performing (the "P") an option. The final step in the A-BAP problem-solving approach focuses on Evaluating (the "E") how the option worked, with a focus on anticipating how the option might impact mood. Adolescents are then asked to practice COPE using Handout 16 "Using COPE" in the upcoming "Test It Out" activity for the week. The therapist should again walk through the steps outlined earlier (i.e., the 5 W's) to maximize the chances that the adolescent will be able to complete the COPE practice.

The remainder of Session 5 involves introducing and practicing with parents supportive ways to communicate with their adolescent using active listening skills as outlined in the teaching guides, Handout 17 "How to Communicate with Support" and Handout 18" Practicing How to Communicate with Support." Parents also are given a "Test It Out" assignment, Handout 19 "Communicating with Support: What Can You Do to Help an Interaction Go Well," to keep track of one time when their communication went well and was supportive and another time when they noted themselves responding less supportively. This is done to increase awareness of what may be automatic response patterns in parents and to begin a discussion with parents about the potential benefit of considering alternate ways of responding to their adolescent.

Session 6: Goal Setting

Session 6 introduces a central skill in the BA approach given the focus on structuring engagement (or reengagement) in activities that are tied to the individual's goals and therefore personally meaningful. Much of this session involves working with the adolescent, but time with parents is also included. With the adolescent, the session focuses on the key concept of how to identify, set, and work to achieve a SMART goal starting with reviewing the Handout 20 teaching guide "Setting SMART Goals." The adolescent is introduced to the concept that "SMART" goals are Specific, Measurable, Appealing, Realistic, and Time-Bound (Doran, 1981; Eggert et al., 1995). Then, the therapist guides an exercise to evaluate and refine a set of goals taking the SMART approach, using the Handout 21 teaching guide "How SMART Is This Goal?" and the Handout 22 worksheet

"Identifying a SMART Goal." The concept of "mini-steps" also is introduced, and the adolescent is asked to consider his or her individual situations (family, school, social, activities) to begin to identify a goal that he or she could work toward and that would contribute to improving his or her situation/mood.

Using the Handout 23 worksheet "Goal Setting," the therapist then works with the adolescent to articulate a SMART goal and identify the mini-steps the adolescent can take to begin to move toward achieving the goal. It is important to allot time for careful attention to naming and refining the goal. Adolescents frequently identify very broad goals (e.g., pass all my classes, lose weight, get a job, graduate from high school) that may take time and many steps to accomplish. Therapists can support the value of the larger, longer-term goal, but it is essential to work with the adolescent to set a series of smaller, achievable goals, and in turn mini-steps toward each goal, so that the adolescent experiences a sense of mastery and success. Parents may need to be included in some of the goal-setting work if the adolescent is focused on a goal that requires parent support and resources.

Drawing on the case examples from Chapter 2, Zach might identify goals of increasing time with his mother or with peers. Given his long history of disappointments with his mother and lack of engagement with friends, each of these "big" goals would need to be molded into something more specific and realistic. Working with him to set a goal of learning about whether more time with his mother was possible given her current circumstances could lead to mini-steps in which he gathered information from his mother, father, and other family members about whether/when they could spend time together, as well as what they could do together that would be satisfying for both mother and son. More specifically, he and the therapist could develop one or two questions about time and availability that Zach could present to his mother, and schedule time to ask her. One obvious barrier to troubleshoot is that his mother may not be available during a time they had scheduled, so he would need to plan, in advance, some backup times. Similarly for peers, Zach might start with a goal of simply finding out whether there were other kids in his school or neighborhood interested in anime and carry out the mini-steps of checking out school clubs/groups, asking around, and looking online for anime groups/contacts in his area. A first mini-step might include looking at a school website or list of social groups. Eva, on the other hand, might set a goal of finishing her senior project, which could be broken down into a more specific "get started" goal, with a series of mini-steps for the week (e.g., spending 30 minutes making a list of possible volunteer opportunities, identifying three that she viewed as feasible and attractive, and developing a phone script to guide her when she called programs to ask about volunteering).

The parent section of this session is designed to include a review of the parents' "Test It Out" assignment from the previous session and more discussion of how parents can show support for their adolescent using the Handout 24 teaching guide "Ways to Support My Adolescent." Parents are asked to identify one of their adolescent's behaviors that they would like to support, then to consider what they might do to support this behavior in an effective manner. The therapist's role is to help parents focus on a behavior that is consistent with the goal of helping the adolescent reengage in rewarding activities as a means of improving his or her mood. Monitoring is presented to parents as a useful way to help us track behaviors we are trying to change. They are given a "Test It Out" assignment using

Handout 25 "Monitoring Support" to monitor or keep track of their supportive behaviors over the course of the coming week. The goal is to highlight all the supportive things parents are already doing, while guiding them to pay attention to shaping their support to the needs of their adolescent.

Session 7: Identifying Barriers

Session 7 continues the focus on goal setting by discussing and normalizing, using the Handout 26 teaching guide "Barriers: Internal versus External," the many barriers that can interfere with making progress toward accomplishing a goal. More specifically, the concept of internal ("not feeling like it," distracted, ruminating) and external (no money, no ride, no "stuff") barriers is reviewed. In this context, it is important to draw out barriers that are meaningful to the adolescent using his or her own examples and to include barriers that might have come up in trying to do (or not do) the "Test It Out" goal-setting assignment (Handout 23: "Goal Setting") from the previous session. Goal-directed versus mood-directed behavior is reviewed again with an eye toward underscoring the importance of recognizing the overpowering pull of one's mood as a barrier to overcome. For instance, Zach's rumination about past disappointments with his mother may have served as a barrier, interfering with his plan to talk with her about her availability. Anticipating and identifying ways to overcome these barriers are critical elements of the activation process.

The next component is to set a new goal and mini-steps for the week to come using Handout 27 "Goals and Barriers" to organize the "Test It Out" activity. This should ideally be the next phase or part of the goal work from the previous week—for Zach, it might be checking out a group or meeting of anime fans he identified the previous week, even if only staying a few minutes or it could be asking someone in his class what he or she knows about the group. For Eva, it could be moving forward, getting her volunteer work set up through the mini-steps of calling three places and using her script. If the goal setting from the previous week did not work out (the adolescent did not follow through, the mini-steps were not useful/effective, the adolescent is unsure about the chosen goal, etc.), then the therapist helps the adolescent to identify a goal in which he or she is more invested, troubleshoots barriers, or revises the goal and mini-steps, while taking the barriers identified this week into account. As in the previous week, careful attention is paid to activity scheduling, and the therapist discusses with the adolescent when each of the mini-steps might be taken given the adolescent's schedule for the week. Barriers are anticipated, and strategies are identified to overcome them as needed.

The session ends with the parent and adolescent talking together about ways in which the parent can show support. The parents' "Test It Out" activity from the previous week is reviewed, and in this meeting the adolescent is asked to let the parent know what kinds of things he or she finds supportive drawing on the Handout 28 teaching guide "Support Ideas," as needed. The goal is to increase communication between the parents and adolescent, and to give the adolescent the opportunity to think about and share what he or she finds supportive. Parents are given a "Test It Out" activity, using Handout 29 "Support Experiment," to identify and track a way to show support over the coming week.

Session 8: Overcoming Avoidance

Session 8 is the last of the more structured skills-teaching sessions. The discussion of barriers is continued, with a focus on avoidance as a specific type of "internal" barrier that commonly gets in the way of taking action toward a goal. The first step is to engage the adolescent in a discussion about the many faces of avoidance and figure out with him or her what avoidance behaviors are barriers using Handout 30 "What Does Avoidance Look Like?" as a teaching guide if helpful. Specific discussion may focus on avoidance behaviors common to adolescents, including brooding (ruminating), bursting (blowing up and becoming emotionally dysregulated), or hibernating (sleeping, isolating). It is important for the therapist to recognize and point out that avoidance can involve positive components, as well as remind the adolescent of the importance of evaluating the function of a behavior rather than its form. For instance, "losing oneself in a book" when parents are arguing may represent positive coping, while reading for hours instead of studying for the next day's math test is likely to be a form of avoidance. Next, it is important to communicate clearly with the adolescent about the nature and function of avoidance. Avoidance "makes sense" because it often provides temporary relief from negative feelings and may feel good in the moment. Over time, however, avoidance can contribute to feelings of distress and depression. As with all the skills presented, the key is to integrate the ideas into the issues and examples that are pertinent to the individual adolescent, helping him or her to identify the ways he or she may be using avoidance to cope with feelings and situations. For some adolescents this will be a straightforward discussion, whereas others may have well-established and comfortable (frequently reinforced) avoidance patterns that may be hard to recognize and change. The goal is to determine whether avoidance is an issue for the adolescent, and if it is, to come up with an example that is pertinent.

Building on the discussion of avoidance, in this session, the therapist also introduces the BA TRAP-TRAC concept (Trigger, Response, Avoidance Pattern–Trigger, Response, Alternative Coping; Jacobson et al., 2001) and focuses on working through an example that fits the adolescent and will make it easier for him or her to see how overcoming avoidance may be useful. The Handout 31 worksheet "Using TRAP-TRAC to Conquer Avoidance and Overcome the Downward Spiral" presents this skill and invites the therapist and the adolescent to work through an example. In so doing, it is important to emphasize that avoidance behaviors can be comfortable (almost automatic!) responses, and working to identify what triggers avoidance and practicing alternative ways of coping will take time and effort. In fact, making such changes may be hard at first and feel more stressful than falling into a familiar pattern of avoidance behavior. This sets the stage for returning the focus to mini-steps and COPE as possible ways to begin to identify alternative coping strategies and for presenting the "Test It Out" activity for the week. Avoidance frequently crops up when adolescents feel anxious, so revisiting the COPE calming strategies may be a useful step before coming up with mini-steps or generating a list of alternative coping strategies. For instance, Rebecca identifies that when conflict or "drama" among her friends get intense (her trigger) she typically shuts down, does not respond to texts or posts, does not do her schoolwork, and even sometimes leaves school or skips classes. In this situation, her therapist could coach her to identify signs of her anxiety rising, use paced breathing to calm herself, then generate a list of alternative coping strategies that include talking to her mother after school, reaching out to a "non-drama queen" friend, and going to the library to do her homework rather than heading home.

The end of the session includes the opportunity for the therapist to check in with parents about their "Test It Out" task from last week—monitoring the number of times they provided support and any observations about how doing so affected the adolescent or themselves (Handout 29: "Support Experiment"). Parents are reminded that the next three sessions will focus on helping the adolescent apply the skills they have learned to unique goals and challenges. Input from parents is requested to help guide the upcoming sessions.

Module 4: Practice (Sessions 9–11)

The same structure (check-in, "Test It Out" review, key concepts/issues, set up of practice for the week to come) is used for the sessions in this section as in other modules. However, the focus of Sessions 9–11 is more individualized. The adolescent and therapist work together to determine the focus and practice assignments for between sessions.

Sessions 9–11: Putting It All Together and Practicing Skills

Session 9 marks a transition from introducing specific concepts and skills to a focus on applying the skills as needed, to addressing the adolescent's key concerns and helping him or her move toward achieving his or her own goals and objectives. After reviewing the "Test It Out" assignment from last session, the therapist introduces the idea that since they have been working together for a couple of months, it might be a good time to review how things are going, think about whether there have been any changes, and identify how the adolescent wants to use his or her remaining time in therapy. If the therapist is in a time-limited practice, this may mean reminding the adolescent how many more sessions the therapist is available to meet, or it can simply be a time to "take stock" and make sure treatment is on a track that is useful to the adolescent. We have used a simple review of weekly mood rating to help visualize changes in mood over time coupled with the Handout 32 worksheet "Taking Stock" as an easy way to review what is going on with the adolescent. It can also be useful to use Handout 2 "How Behavioral Activation Works for You" from Session 1 to revisit what was going on when the adolescent came into treatment, think about what is different now, and recognize what is currently contributing to or helping to reduce negative feelings.

The adolescent is then supported while he or she thinks through priorities for the next (or remaining) period of treatment and translates these into an action plan with a SMART goal and mini-steps. At this point in treatment the adolescent may have already identified a goal on which he or she is still actively working, so continuing to work toward that goal by articulating and trying out mini-steps with attention to overcoming barriers and avoidance might be indicated. However, this is a time to make sure that the issues that are important to the adolescent are being actively addressed and to incorporate skills as needed to accomplish this task.

The "Test It Out" task for this session and the next two sessions is developed in collaboration with the adolescent via the process of identifying what the adolescent wants to focus on, then outlining what kind of activity will be needed using Handout 33 "Developing an Action Plan," and using Handout 34 "Action Plan" to plan specific times when they will take the mini-steps identified. For instance, Zach may choose to continue to work on his relationship with his mother by using goal-directed versus mood-directed strategies to arrange times for them to be together and also practice making the most of any good moments he has with her. Eva, on the other hand, may want to branch out from her focus on getting her senior project done to focus on making new friends—which might mean helping her manage the barrier of feeling anxious in social interactions by outlining things she can say to enter a social group or ways to focus her attention on the other people rather than worrying only about what she will say next. Sessions 10 and 11 are geared to ongoing work in support of the adolescent's goals, always with a focus on increasing active engagement in activities that are rewarding and fostering a sense of mastery and competence. In these sessions the therapist can review any material presented in earlier sessions, practice skills in session, and set up practice experiments with the adolescent.

Module 5: Moving Forward (Session 12)

Session 12: Relapse Prevention and Saying Good-Bye

This session follows the same format as prior sessions, although its focus is on summing up treatment and developing a plan that will help the adolescent cope effectively with ongoing and future stressors, without an exacerbation of depressive symptoms. Only one new concept is presented within the context of relapse prevention, namely, that "slips," such as feeling depressed or unmotivated in response to a disappointment, are common but temporary and need to be recognized, and that skills learned in the A-BAP process can be used to overcome these setbacks. The therapist then works with the adolescent to walk through the types of stressors and triggers they can anticipate and identify strategies they can use as they plan how to handle triggers and cope with problems that are bound to come up using the Handout 35 worksheet "Doing What Works." It is also important to review with both the adolescent and parents indicators of possible relapse, such as persistence of symptoms, interference with the ability to participate in school and favorite activities, as well as thoughts of self-harm/suicide, as these indicators would suggest that the adolescent is not just having a "bad day/week" but may need to consider returning for additional treatment. Even though this might be the last therapy session, it is important for the therapist to end his or her time with the adolescent walking through the "Test It Out" practice that he or she can continue to work on and refine on his or her own over time. Troubleshoot barriers to continuing these efforts and be sure to comment on the progress made, the effort extended, and the adolescents' ability to continue this work without a therapist or coach, with the remainder of the session devoted to who they can turn to for help and support.

The A-BAP manual suggests ending this session with a review of progress and Handout 35 "Doing What Works" with parents. This, of course, will vary with the treatment context, adolescents' needs, and family circumstances.

Note on Timing of Termination

Although the A-BAP is designed to be a 12- to 14-session intervention delivered approximately once a week, when to end therapy clearly depends on the needs of each adolescent. More specifically, an adolescent could be scheduled to terminate the week she and her boyfriend break up, or the week that his grandmother, to whom he is very close, passes away. In the A-BAP, therapists are encouraged to take heed and to adjust and plan accordingly. The therapist may choose to delay termination for a couple of weeks and/or spread out sessions in the latter part of treatment to every other week, depending on the needs of the adolescent and the policies and procedures in one's respective clinic. For example, Gina, a 15-year-old girl, was coming to the end of her A-BAP treatment just as she was also getting ready to transition into a new school. The previous year she had attended a prestigious private school and had come to the painful decision that she just did not fit in and would perhaps be happier attending her neighborhood public school. This decision was fraught with challenges for Gina. Although Gina was very bright, she felt out of place at this private school given her socioeconomic background, and with her depression had struggled to keep up with the demanding workload. Gina had requested to start the new academic year at a public school, and although it went against her parents' hopes and desires, Gina's parents were in support of her decision. Although Gina's treatment was coming to an end, it grew increasingly clear to her therapist that Gina not only had a high level of anxiety about stepping into a new school and not knowing anyone but that this transition would also be crucial to setting the stage for a successful high school experience. A decision was made, therefore, to stretch out Gina's termination process. Appointments were made to coincide with the first week of school and again 2 weeks later, with a plan to continue to consider the need for additional appointments. Although Gina had a great deal of anxiety the first week of school, she used the skills she had learned through A-BAP; did not fall back into patterns of avoidance; and, with good planning, navigated the transition successfully. Upon returning for her second follow-up visit, Gina was in excellent spirits, shared that she had met some new friends, and was feeling positive about her decision to transition to her neighborhood school. With this, a collaborative decision was made among Gina, her parents, and the therapist to terminate treatment, with the option to call for additional support, if needed.

Integration of BA with Other Therapeutic Strategies

Recent evidence, as reviewed in Chapter 1, suggests the usefulness of a modularized approach to treatment that encourages use of specific evidence-based treatment strategies "as needed" to address problem areas as they arise in the course of treatment. While the A-BAP provides a session-by-session structure, therapists can readily incorporate components of A-BAP into a broader CBT or IPT treatment. We make the following suggestions, however, when therapists use the material in this fashion. First, keep in mind that BA is a principle-driven therapy that is tailored for each adolescent based on the behavioral assessment and functional analysis. Furthermore, implementation of strategies developed in BA or in A-BAP specifically should be used only when they fit with a comprehensive case conceptualization or formulation (Eells, 2007). In other words, we do not advocate doing "a little BA" here and there as the need arises. Rather, maintenance factors in depression, such as avoidance behavior, mood-directed behavior, and general disengagement, having been identified as problematic for a given adolescent client, can be addressed using modules from the A-BAP. These would be planned according to the case formulation. Persons (2008) suggests that therapists develop a problem list during the initial assessment stage of therapy and plan interventions that have been validated to deal with specific problems. The main ingredients of BA are activity monitoring and scheduling, identifying potentially reinforcing activities by articulating goals that are important to or highly valued by the adolescent, and identifying barriers to activation and addressing them. One particular barrier to activation that is addressed in A-BAP is avoidance behavior. In the case conceptualization, when the function of the adolescent's behavior is identified as avoidance, BA strategies can be planned.

Second, when therapists believe that elements of BA will be helpful in treatment, but that the case conceptualization is mostly consistent with CBT or IPT, planning in advance a structure that would logically make use of the A-BAP modules or sessions would also be helpful. Homework is standard practice in these treatments, so anticipating the use of A-BAP, the therapist may frame homework as "Test It Out" from the start of treatment. This allows the therapist to incorporate a session outline and handouts from A-BAP with relative ease, without confusing the adolescent with a sudden change in structure. Components from A-BAP that could be readily integrated into ongoing CBT or IPT care include activity monitoring and scheduling, identification of reinforcing behaviors (Handout 12: "Pump You Up, Bring You Down" activities), identification of barriers (Handout 26: "Barriers: Internal versus External"), and developing alternative coping strategies (Handout 31: "Using TRAP-TRAC to Conquer Avoidance and Overcome the Downward Spiral").

It may well be that in the future of empirically supported treatments, strategies to address specific transdiagnostic problems will be the norm rather than the use of entire protocols. This would certainly be in keeping with the idiographic nature of behavior therapy that addresses behaviors rather than diagnoses. Practically, therapists are often faced with clients who do not meet criteria for only one diagnosis, or they have problems that a particular protocol does not adequately address. The modular nature of A-BAP is ideally suited to be used either as a full treatment package or the components can be used as needed based on the case formulation.

CHAPTER 4

Management of Treatment Challenges within the A-BAP Approach

The A-BAP approach provides a theoretically based and well-defined set of strategies for working with adolescents who are struggling with depression. Each adolescent, however, presents with his or her unique needs and circumstances, and as a result, challenging situations undoubtedly arise over the course of treatment. Although it is not possible to outline all treatment challenges, some are common when working with depressed adolescents. This chapter reviews common treatment challenges and offers strategies for handling and managing them within the A-BAP model. These challenges, which are viewed as a routine part of working with adolescents and families, typically fall into three main categories: (1) engagement, (2) escalation of distress and symptoms, and (3) family and/or environmental circumstances.

Engagement

Issues concerning therapeutic engagement come in all shapes, sizes, and packages; include a wide variety of variables; and are common to all forms of psychotherapy. The interrelated list of issues that comprise the construct of engagement, include challenges with (1) initial engagement/rapport building, (2) regular attendance, (3) homework completion, (4) motivation to change, and (5) agreement between therapist and adolescent concerning treatment targets. In our practice and application of the BA approach to treatment, we have seen and been challenged by all of these concerns at some point in time. Although we will go through each of the categories outlined earlier and offer practical information regarding such treatment challenges, it should also be noted that, as discussed in Chapter 1, the A-BAP draws on evidence-supported techniques (Naar-King & Suarez, 2011; Nock & Ferriter, 2005) to enhance engagement regardless of the issue/concern. In general, it is our hope that BA therapists always adopt an open, interested, and authentic stance that allows the therapist to understand and validate the engagement concern, while simultaneously trying to evoke change talk and an experimental attitude. As noted previously, this includes the use of *evocation, collaboration,* and core MI communication strategies, such as *open-ended questions, affirmations, reflective listening,* and *summaries* (Miller & Rollnick, 2002).

Challenges with Initial Engagement/Rapport Building

As is universal in all therapies, the therapeutic alliance in BA cannot be underestimated. Pellerin, Costa, Weems, and Dalton (2010) estimate that at least 50% of youth who begin treatment do not complete it. One factor that undoubtedly underlies this statistic centers on the therapeutic alliance. In general, research has highlighted the importance of a number of variables in increasing the therapeutic alliance with adolescents, including perceptions of the therapist as warm, respectful, open, trusting, and offering guidance (Shirk & Karver, 2003; Martin, Romas, Medford, Leffert, & Hatcher, 2006). Some authors have further noted the inherent challenges in developing a therapeutic alliance with adolescents, specifically, given the adolescents' need to develop independence and differentiate from authority figures (Eltz, Shirk, & Sarlin, 1995).

As highlighted in Chapter 3, in the A-BAP, efforts are made in the first sessions to ensure that therapist and adolescent get off to a good start. More specifically, adolescents and their parents are given clear information about the structure and nature of the treatment; the roles of the therapist, adolescent and parent(s); and what to expect as treatment progresses—all factors that have been found to promote initial engagement and attendance (Nock & Ferriter, 2005). In addition, therapists pay particularly close attention to "hearing" and "understanding" the adolescent's story from his or her perspective. Although the A-BAP emphasizes this more in the first two sessions, as the therapist works to understand the adolescent's history, he or she must remain sensitive to the potential vulnerability in the therapeutic alliance over time. Specifically, the therapist must carefully monitor issues related to the therapeutic relationship, taking the requisite amount of time required by each adolescent throughout therapy to keep the therapeutic alliance in good order. Although the A-BAP is quite structured and prescriptive at times, therapists should never feel a need to push forward in the face of jeopardizing the therapeutic alliance. One way that this is emphasized in BA centers on the therapist's role as a "coach" who offers structure and guidance in a warm manner (Martin et al., 2006), while allowing the adolescent the opportunity to achieve developmental needs related to independence and differentiating from authority figures (Eltz et al., 1995). Failure to maintain a coaching stance in BA not only jeopardizes the therapeutic alliance, but it also further risks the structure of the program, which highlights partnering with the adolescent and encouraging the practice of concept-related skills.

Challenges with Regular Attendance

Poor and/or spotty attendance makes the conduct of any therapy challenging, and it is no different in BA. As with most therapies, a lack of attendance or intermittent attendance frequently leads to situations in which it is challenging, if not impossible, to gain treatment momentum. One strategy known to enhance ongoing attendance (Nock & Ferriter, 2005) and built into the A-BAP is the inclusion of time with the parent(s) (by phone or in person) to provide support, get ongoing input, and bolster coping skills. When a pattern of poor or intermittent attendance has been realized, however, the A-BAP therapist is encouraged to approach and address intermittent attendance as a problem and attempt to understand it in the context of a functional analysis. More specifically, the therapist is encouraged to work with the adolescent, and perhaps even his or her parent(s), to understand the antecedents to the behavior and the function the behavior serves, essentially assessing and working to overcome barriers to treatment—a practice element frequently used in engagement interventions (Becker et al., 2015). It has been our experience that the function behind intermittent treatment attendance can vary a great deal from adolescent to adolescent. For some adolescents, particularly as they begin to feel better, therapy becomes burdensome and is perceived by them to interfere with efforts toward activation. For others, intermittent or spotty attendance may reflect other struggles. For instance, it may be that the adolescent was never "on board" with the treatment in the first place, and treatment may have been something the adolescent's parent(s) wanted. Alternatively, the adolescent may have no interest in giving up his or her identity as a depressed adolescent, and because treatment challenges this "identity," the adolescent is not interested in continuing on the journey. Or it may be that the adolescent is not finding relief from the treatment and is struggling to find the motivation to attend. Regardless of what the function may be, the therapist is encouraged to address it directly with the adolescent and his or her parent(s) in an effort to problem-solve and get the treatment back on track.

While we ultimately view poor or spotty attendance as a problem to be solved jointly by therapist and adolescent, the therapist needs to actively reach out and help to problem-solve. The discussion should include a functional analysis of the behavior, with ample opportunity for the adolescent to speak honestly about the process of therapy without concern about reprisal. In addition, this discussion must also include some consideration of the idea that it is difficult to gain treatment momentum without regular attendance and that, at least in some cases, spotty attendance can reinforce beliefs that therapy is not helpful or should be used only in the event of a "crisis." With that said, it is the therapist's job to listen carefully and problem-solve with the adolescent in a flexible manner. For example, it might mean that an agreement is made to alternate between in-person and remote sessions (e.g., skype). Likewise, it might mean that the therapist and adolescent agree to an alternative, but consistent, therapy schedule that could include every other week attendance, with off weeks used for preferred activities. Failure to address intermittent attendance in therapy altogether will inevitably result in ongoing frustration for the therapist, adolescent, or both. An example of how such a discussion might take place is as follows:

> THERAPIST: Before we get started today, I want to make sure we touch base on a few things. I have not seen you in a couple of weeks and this has been a pretty consistent pattern—I see you for 2 or 3 weeks in a row, and then there is a session or two that is missed, and then I see you again, and so forth. It sometimes seems

that as you start to feel better, therapy becomes less important, and then when something does not go so well, therapy seems more important. I am wondering if I am accurate about that or if you have other thoughts and ideas about it all?

PATIENT: I guess I just do not see the point in coming if everything is going okay. Since I started coming here, I have been doing a lot better. I mean I still have my "ups and downs," but for the most part, especially lately, it seems like it does not make a lot of sense to come all the time.

THERAPIST: Well . . . I certainly understand how it can feel that way. Maybe we should talk about it, however, because I think we might see it really differently.

PATIENT: Okay. I just really don't see the point in coming when everything has been going smoothly. I mean . . . I just don't really see what it is I would talk about.

THERAPIST: I can totally see why it might seem that there is nothing to talk about in those situations. I guess I view therapy a bit differently. I think when things are going really smoothly for you, it offers us a time to talk about what skills you have been using that have helped in this regard. It also allows us to continue to learn about new skills and provides us with a time when we can compare and contrast different situations. For example, you might come in and tell me about an argument you had with your parents and yet for some reason, it did not bother you in the same way it has bothered you at other times. It would be important for us to look at that and identify what was different and how you might have felt after you tried something that you learned in therapy. In a way, I think we can use therapy to learn about what helped a situation to "go right" versus "go wrong." By virtue of learning about this and comparing and contrasting, sometimes it can give you really important information moving forward. Otherwise, you might just be coming to therapy in times that are more like a "crisis," and if we are only ever focused on the "crisis," we will not have the same opportunity to learn about all the important things you are doing to help things go more smoothly for yourself. Related to this, it might also be the case that if you come regularly, you might be able to complete therapy sooner, because you are consistently working on the issues that originally brought you in and building on the things you have learned. Does that make sense?

PATIENT: I guess that makes sense.

THERAPIST: I have an idea. How about you call me if you find yourself thinking about canceling a session? We can talk about the pros and cons of coming in or not and I can remind you of how therapy can be useful even when you are feeling pretty good.

PATIENT: Okay, that sounds good. Also, even though I like you and everything, I like the idea that I might be able to finish therapy sooner and not have to come back at all.

THERAPIST: I like that idea for you as well!

Challenges with Homework Completion

It is not uncommon in behaviorally based therapies, such as A-BAP, for therapists to ask youth to engage in "out-of-session" homework activities between appointments (Kazantzis, Deane, & Ronan, 2000). This strategy has long been used and, when completed, is a useful one for skill consolidation, gaining an understanding of trouble spots with regard to the adolescent's understanding of material, ensuring the generalization of concepts taught to the adolescent, and guaranteeing that the adolescent will engage with the material at some point between sessions. Although there are many benefits to the concept of "homework," the fact remains that many adolescents, for whatever reason, cannot seem to complete it. Once again, it presents the therapist with an opportunity to attempt to understand barriers to homework completion through a functional analysis. As is the case with regard to poor attendance, a range of variables may explain poor homework completion, including, but not limited to, low motivation, lack of clarity about what is being asked, a desire to keep painful realizations at bay between sessions, and/or a lack of interest in changing or getting better. The therapist must also remain open to the possibility that he or she has played an important role in the adolescent's poor homework completion. More specifically, some therapists inadvertently send a message about homework, either downplaying its importance or apologizing for assigning it, both of which likely serve as barriers to its completion. As there is no one "cause" of lack of compliance with homework, it is inherent upon the therapist to understand it in a manner that ultimately moves the treatment forward. In so doing, the therapist is strongly encouraged to remain committed to communicating the importance of homework—never failing to take time both to talk through the homework to ensure that it is clear and that it fits the adolescent's needs. In addition, the therapist must review the previous week's homework assignment in each session and, if need be, guide in-session completion. Failure to do so reinforces the patient's poor compliance with homework completion, because it ultimately sends the message "It's okay that you did not complete it—we weren't going to use it in our treatment anyway." In fact, this is one reason why homework review is a part of every session outline in A-BAP. Whether completed out of session and brought in, or completed in-session, homework offers the therapist an opportunity to assess the adolescent's understanding of therapeutic material and allow for reteaching of material, if necessary. It also provides the therapist with good material on which to build the teaching of new concepts. Throughout, the therapist is encouraged to send the message that "practice makes perfect," and practicing skills and strategies in times of little stress will increase the likelihood that they will be useful when they are truly needed.

Outside of reinforcing the importance of homework in the BA model, therapists are also strongly encouraged to structure the homework assignment in a manner that increases the likelihood of completion. Much like the therapist would structure a process of goal setting, the focus would be on the following:

1. What is the assignment?
2. How long will it take?

3. Given how long it will take, when can the adolescent commit to doing it?
4. What are the barriers that might get in the way?
5. Knowing the barriers, what countermeasures can the adolescent take to complete the assignment?

As is the case with goal setting, the more structure the therapist can offer around homework completion, the greater the likelihood it will happen.

Challenges with Motivation to Change

A small subset of depressed adolescents appears to lack motivation to change. This often seems to be a function of the youth taking on an identity as a depressed individual. As uncomfortable as the depression may be, the youth seems to recognize that his or her depression has put him or her in a position of perhaps being a philosophical, reflective, and deep-thinking individual—qualities and characteristics that the adolescent may value and by virtue of this, may be reticent to give up. More specifically, some adolescents seem to believe that getting better and "giving up" their depression will lead to a fundamental change in their identity and who they are as a person; potentially, they even fear that should they give up their depression, they will be devoid of a list of personal qualities on which they have come to place high value. Similarly, other adolescents feel that if they give up their depression, they will be giving up life as they have known it and feel anxious about the "unknowns" that lie ahead (e.g., will others respond to them differently, etc.), particularly if they have been struggling with depression for a long time or during the majority of their adolescent years.

As is the case in just about any therapy, MI techniques are an excellent way to manage discussions related to this, with a particular focus on what is needed to just take a small step and "try something on for size," without having to take what feels to be a drastic step and "give up" the depression completely. Related to this, the challenge for the BA therapist is to help the adolescent find opportunities that allow him or her to maintain an identity as a philosophical, reflective, and deep-thinking individual, while also getting activated. This is exemplified in the case of Zach, the adolescent boy introduced in Chapter 2, who "identified" a great deal with his depression, and as depressed as he could honestly say he was, there was something very threatening to him about giving it up. While he had impeccable attendance at his therapy appointments, he openly criticized the treatment, saying it "wasn't working" or that assignments seemed "silly, unhelpful, and trivial." Instead of arguing with him about this, Zach's therapist took the approach of appealing to his view of himself as a smart, deep-thinking, artistic, and creative young man. Specifically, Zach's therapist shared that while there was no guarantee that the A-BAP approach would be helpful for him, perhaps his engagement in the treatment and with the materials could be helpful to other youth. To this end, Zach's therapist asked him to "get activated" by using his artistic talents and creativity to critique worksheets and homework assignments constructively, in a manner that might ultimately help to make the treatment more useful and effective for other adolescents. Zach bought into this approach and weekly offered his therapist information on what he thought of each strategy, worksheet, and homework assignment, essentially sharing a list of ideas for how each could be improved. Interestingly, in order to do so, Zach had to engage in the process of trying each strategy, and although he continued to share that he thought they were silly, he nevertheless gradually became more activated. Never once was it suggested that he needed to give up his reflective and deep thinking, or his artistic and creative side. Instead, he was simply challenged to use them in the context of getting activated.

Lack of motivation to change can also be buried in the context of rumination. As detailed in some of our earlier work (McCauley, Schloredt, Gudmundsen, Martell, & Dimidjian, 2015), rumination is a construct that is frequently associated with depression (Nolen-Hoeksema, 2000), and has two distinct subtypes: brooding and reflective problem solving (Treynor, Gonzalez, & Nolen-Hoeksema, 2003), which are associated with differential outcomes. If an adolescent engages in rumination, it is of utmost importance for the BA therapist to understand this in context. More specifically, research evidence would suggest that "brooding" rumination is associated with more negative outcomes related to depressive symptoms and disengagement coping, whereas rumination associated with "reflecting" is associated with more positive outcomes (Burwell & Shirk, 2007; Lo, Ho, & Hollon, 2008; Treynor et al., 2003).

For example, consider Alison, a 15-year-old girl with a long history of engaging in rumination, particularly with regard to her social relationships. She would spend hours anticipating social interactions with her friends, as well as going over and over her interactions after the fact. Gradually, Alison was receptive to engaging in a functional behavior analysis of this repetitive thinking behavior, even though she insisted it was both helpful and just a part of who she is as a person. Through assessment, we learned that when her mood was low, Alison's thinking behavior involved brooding and getting quite stuck on factors that were out of her control—conversations that had already happened, responses made by her friend, or her own emotional responses in the moment. She would get stuck on these thoughts for hours, going over the past events that did not go well in an effort to ensure that it never happened again; however, the result was her stewing in the negative past and becoming increasingly pessimistic about her ability to behave differently in a similar situation in the future. Additionally, this would make her feel more down and irritable. Alternatively, when Alison's mood was neutral to high, not only did she engage in such thinking less frequently, but she also seemed better able to reflect. She was able to let go and accept things that did not go well, as well as acknowledge the limits of what she could or not do. And she was able to move on to other things, whether it was homework or investing her energy in other relationships. Alison learned the typical triggers and patterns to her rumination and agreed to rate her mood when these situations happened. If her mood was low (4 or lower on a scale of 1 to 10), she would engage in a "pump you up" activity in an effort to boost her mood and prevent brooding. If her mood was a 5 or higher, Alison was allowed to engage in thinking, but she found it helpful to set a timer in order to limit it to 5 minutes and prevent a downward spiral.

The example of Alison highlights the challenges that rumination poses to BA treatment and how easily rumination can equate to a lack of motivation to change. What is of utmost importance here is the therapist's role in completing a functional analysis of the ruminative behavior with the adolescent, such that it can be recognized by the adolescent for what it is. With that comes the important task of helping the adolescent identify the rumination in the moment (e.g., recognizing that the adolescent is in a TRAP—trigger, response, avoidance pattern) and overcoming the rumination by identifying alternative coping strategies or behaviors, in this case "pump you up" activities, as a way to get back on track (e.g., TRAC—trigger, response, alternative coping) and manage the behavior over time.

Challenges with Agreement Concerning Treatment Targets

One potentially complicating factor in the treatment of adolescents is that they often do not self-identify and present for treatment; rather, the process is driven by a parent or caregiver. To this end, therapists can sometimes find themselves treating adolescents who do not fundamentally believe that there is a problem and/or perhaps do not agree with the treatment targets they are given. These cases are always challenging for therapists, regardless of the treatment modality they are using. The same is true with regard to A-BAP. In our practice, we have run across this situation on several occasions—parents reporting a history strongly suggestive and consistent with depression and adolescents vehemently denying it in favor of some other terminology and/or some other treatment target. When such is the case and the adolescent can "own" the idea that something is not right and he or she might benefit from treatment, we have always taken the simple approach of using the language the adolescent uses to identify what is not working well. A classic example of this is the case of Peter, identified earlier in this book (Chapter 2). Although Peter was not ready or willing to admit to being depressed, he was open to treatment by virtue of the fact that he felt disconnected from others and could recognize that he desired more of a social life but was completely unsure of how to achieve it. In his case, Peter's therapist was careful not to use the word *depression* or push the idea with him, but instead focused on the words Peter used and capitalized on his goal of desiring more activity with friends but feeling stuck with regard to how to make that happen.

In alignment with dimensional models of classification (Helzer et al., 2006; Kraemer, 2007), it has always been our stance that it is not so much what one chooses to call "it" as long as there is an agreed-upon therapeutic target and willingness to engage in the process. Pushing an adolescent to accept the treatment target of depression really serves no purpose and potentially only alienates him or her from engaging in any type of treatment. Instead, focusing on the terminology preferred by the adolescent sets up a collaborative dynamic that may ultimately allow the adolescent to view his or her struggles differently over time and, more importantly, helps him or her feel validated throughout the treatment process, which in turn enhances the therapeutic alliance and relationship.

Summary Regarding Engagement

In summary, there are many issues that threaten or pose challenges to engagement, and we have only addressed a few of the more common challenges we have come across in our use of the A-BAP. While we have outlined a number of potential engagement challenges here, our list, and how to manage them, is not exhaustive. In a recent study, Becker and colleagues (2015) examined three domains of treatment engagement, namely, attendance, adherence (e.g., session participation, homework completion), and cognitive preparation (e.g., expectations about roles, motivation for change), in relation to treatment outcomes, and highlighted a list of practice elements that were common in studies with successful outcomes. These practice elements included many practices that we commonly engage in as part of the A-BAP—ongoing assessment, psychoeducation and managing expectations about roles and services, assessing and understanding barriers to treatment, and assigning homework—all of which have been discussed or outlined elsewhere. The bottom line is that challenges inevitably emerge in any treatment program, and in order to try to effect positive outcomes, the therapist must not only be prepared for them but must also plan for them and have a good sense of how to manage them, in an effort to keep adolescents engaged and moving forward in treatment.

Escalation of Distress and Symptoms

In Chapter 2, we discussed youth for whom A-BAP is *not* appropriate and problems for which a therapist would want to think about alternative evidence-based treatments; in Chapter 5, we will discuss applications of BA with other clinical samples of youth for whom BA is an appropriate match. The focus here centers on the challenges presented by problems that are present in the context of an escalation of distress or symptoms, including (1) "crisis of the week" scenarios, (2) high-risk behaviors, and (3) acuity (i.e., suicidality).

Challenges with Managing "Crisis of the Week" Scenarios

In any psychotherapeutic treatment program, "crises" that occur "week in and week out" have the potential to derail the therapeutic process and make it challenging for therapy to move forward in a productive manner. Instead of the therapist and adolescent being able to build on strategies from week to week, the focus of the therapy turns toward managing the "crisis *du jour*." While there are some adolescents who do face an occasional "crisis," there are others for whom "crises" dominate their clinical picture. The challenge for the A-BAP therapist is to recognize the frequency and pattern of such "crises" and manage them accordingly. The infrequent crisis that does *not* appear to represent an ongoing issue or avoidance behavior can be managed quite differently than an ongoing pattern of crisis behavior that ultimately interferes with and/or derails treatment. In the former, the importance of therapist flexibility and attention to the adolescent's immediate needs cannot be underestimated. As noted elsewhere, a therapist may pull forward an unplanned module, as needed, in the context of the "crisis" that the adolescent is presenting. At the same time, it has been our experience that as a therapist becomes more skilled and adept with the BA model, he or she can literally take almost any content with which the adolescent might present and find a way to adapt the lesson to that content. In the event of a crisis, it is not unusual for therapists to abandon their treatment plans to address the crisis. While safety in any crisis situation must be ensured, the A-BAP therapist works with the adolescent to apply related A-BAP treatment strategies to manage the crisis that the adolescent presents. If "crises," however, become frequent and represent a pattern of behavior, a different challenge lies in front of the BA therapist. Specifically, crises that occur with regularity can be defined as "avoidance behavior." The idea here is that the crisis, or rather a series of crises, serves to switch the focus of therapy away from moving the treatment plan forward. In this situation, the therapist should and must address the behavior that has essentially turned into the "elephant in the room." Consistent with everything in BA, the behavior should be framed in the context of a functional analysis, and the therapist should invite the adolescent to look at it, which essentially serves to refocus the adolescent on the treatment plan at hand. If not addressed, spotty attendance might crop up, given the implicit message that therapy functions as a way to solve crises rather than as a way to proactively learn skills.

An example of a "crisis of the week" scenario occurred with Josh, a 16-year-old boy, who lived with his mother and older brother and had not seen his father in several years. Josh had high aspirations for himself, and desired, more than anything, to be a successful lawyer, because he felt this would allow him to be able to provide his mother with a comfortable way of life. Despite Josh's desires, he was struggling to get up and out of bed each morning and to school on time. As he started the A-BAP protocol, he presented each week with some sort of crisis that he felt needed immediate attention. One week, his crisis centered on concerns related to his mother's health; another week, his crisis centered on news that he was failing Language Arts; and the next week, his crisis centered on the stress related to his father reaching out to him after several years of being disengaged. Each week, Josh's therapist was challenged to apply A-BAP modules to the material Josh presented, while advancing treatment forward. Related to this, Josh's therapist felt comfortable conceptualizing with Josh that each of these issues was connected to his depression and helped him to understand them in the context of the A-BAP model by drawing links between these situations, his moods, and the activities he was choosing.

During his fourth week of treatment, Josh's mother called approximately 2 hours prior to his session and shared that Josh had received an emergency expulsion from school for making veiled threats about having a weapon in the context of a verbal argument with a peer in the cafeteria. She noted that the school had taken Josh's threat so seriously that they contacted the police, who then called her because they needed to search the family home. Josh's mother was extremely worried about Josh and unsure about what his behavior meant. It was only his fourth week in the protocol, and prior to this, Josh and his therapist had worked through a different crisis each week. Although, in previous sessions, Josh's therapist had felt comfortable applying the lesson at hand to Josh's concerns and was able to move treatment forward effectively according to the original treatment plan, this seemed quite different. First and foremost, Josh's therapist felt that he would need to abandon the session plan (Introducing Consequences of Behavior), at least in part, to complete a risk assessment and potentially seek appropriate resources (e.g., hospitalization) if need be. Second, the therapist was noticing a pattern of behavior in which each week seemed to bring a new crisis of sorts, and Josh did not seem to be applying what he had previously learned in session to the issues at hand. With this information in mind, Josh's therapist took some time prior to the session to seek consultation with a BA colleague to outline a plan moving forward. Specifically, the plan was to address the "crisis" today by completing a risk assessment and, depending on assessment results, either seek hospitalization or move forward with treatment, specifically by applying the planned session material—functional analysis—to the crisis at hand. Then, based on the information gathered in the functional behavior analysis, the therapist would consider pulling forward BA concepts and strategies related to problem solving (Session 5: Problem Solving) to address school reentry, as well as to understand the nuances of "avoidance behavior," including the concept of "bursting" (Session 8: Overcoming Avoidance). Because this was a lot to cover in one session, Josh's therapist and his colleague discussed the need to focus on immediate concerns related to safety and school reentry, then consider the need to address the possibility of a different pattern of "avoidance behavior" related to ongoing crises by scheduling an extra appointment that week or highlighting it as the focus of the next session.

When Josh arrived for the appointment, he was tearful and quite remorseful. He expressed great fear that he had "ruined" things for himself and would not be allowed to live down his actions with the principal, teachers, and the other kids at school. He also expressed deep frustration with the boy he had threatened, noting that he was tired of "being teased" and wishing that school personnel would recognize this boy for the "bully" that he was. In taking the time to do a risk assessment, as well as a functional analysis of Josh's behavior, the therapist felt confident that Josh did not pose a real threat to his classmate, others at school, or himself, and that his actions were driven by feeling overwhelmed and saddened by the comments of the other young man and "bursting" in the form of a threat in an effort to get this young man to back off and leave him alone. With this, the therapist not only taught Josh about the concept of functional analysis but also introduced ideas related to problem solving and avoidance, namely, discussing "bursting" in the context of a need to make this boy stop, as opposed to problem solving his way through the situation and rationally thinking about his options and choosing one to try and evaluate (COPE). They also used the COPE approach to figure out next steps Josh could take to sort things out at school, and agreed that he would contact his counselor right after session and ask for help in working with the principal. This plan was reviewed with Josh's mother at the end of the session, and she was on board and willing to reach out to Josh's principal. Toward the end of the session, the therapist hypothesized about a pattern of "avoidance behavior" through repeated crises, and Josh and the therapist started a discussion that they ultimately agreed they would pick up during the next session.

At the start of the next session, Josh noted that while all sorts of events had happened, they were primarily indicative of his ongoing struggles with depression and that none was really a "crisis," just situations in which he needed to learn to apply skills in order to cope. Having admitted this, he sheepishly and embarrassingly shared a belief that he "thought" that the process of therapy was about coming and "venting" about how "bad things are" rather than working on strategies for ongoing coping and managing. This provided a perfect opportunity for the therapist to reiterate information about BA roles and expectations and gave Josh and his mother an opportunity to recommit to the process they had started.

Challenges with Managing High-Risk Behaviors

Much like "crisis of the week" scenarios and how these scenarios often represent "avoidance behavior," the same is true with regard to managing high-risk behaviors, including but not limited to self-harming behaviors such as cutting or burning, sexting, sexual risk taking, and substance use. At first recognition, the adolescent and therapist should examine the behavior in the context of BA tools, specifically, functional behavior analysis, and understand what the behavior means and how it relates to the adolescent's ongoing struggles with depression. How the therapist manages the behavior from there centers on the adolescent's response and takes the form of a three-pronged approach. If the adolescent can respond to this discussion with a commitment to examine and work on the behavior in the context of skills learned through BA, the behavior can simply become an active treatment target that is prioritized and monitored. As part of this discussion, the therapist and adolescent should collaboratively examine and understand whether the behavior serves as a form of "avoidance," and if so, the therapist should support the adolescent in understanding it in the TRAP-TRAC algorithm. The real challenge comes in situations in which (1) the behavior continues to escalate (despite it being an active treatment target) and the therapist is not seeing the needed symptom change or (2) the adolescent does not see the destructiveness of the behavior and how it is inconsistent with BA treatment goals, and cannot commit to working on the issue with a goal of giving up the behavior. Both situations require a therapist to make a determination as to whether an augmentation strategy involving components of other treatment needs to be pulled into the A-BAP approach. For example, in the event of increased escalation, the therapist may choose to pull in components of DBT focused on distress tolerance; in the event of the latter, the therapist may attempt to stimulate motivation toward healthy behavior using MI techniques, all with the goal of the behavior becoming a treatment target that is then monitored. If behavioral escalation continues or the adolescent continues to struggle to see the destructiveness of the behavior, the therapist must then make a determination as to whether another approach altogether is indicated.

Challenges with Managing Suicidality

Consistent with any treatment for depression, it is likely that suicidal ideation and/or behavior will become an issue from time to time. As noted elsewhere, part of the BA protocol involves assessing suicide risk on a weekly basis. More specifically, we recommend the use of a questionnaire to get a quick assessment of symptoms, including suicidality, such as the PHQ-9 (Richardson et al., 2010; see Chapter 2). Additionally, we recommend a more in-depth look at suicidality once every 3 weeks or so (see Chapter 2; we used the critical items from the SIQ [Reynolds, 1987]). Outside of these approaches, however, is the issue of managing suicidality if or when it becomes an issue. As always, the therapist and adolescent should attempt to understand suicidality collaboratively in the context of a functional behavioral analysis: the context in which it emerges, the triggering factors, and what the adolescent does when thoughts of suicide, or wanting to die, present. Much like other high-risk behaviors (e.g., sexting, cutting oneself, substance use), what a BA therapist ultimately does with suicidality depends on its chronicity and severity, the functional behavior analysis, and the adolescent's willingness to examine and work on it in the context of skills learned through BA. Specifically, if the adolescent endorses suicidal ideation with no plan and no intention to act, a safety plan should be developed; then, suicidality can be prioritized and treated as any other treatment target with monitoring that is ongoing, particularly if the adolescent is willing to work on it in context of BA treatment, applying skills learned through BA to situations in which the thoughts and feelings arise. Alternatively, if the therapist feels there is acute, serious, and persistent risk, consideration of more intensive care is indicated, including the possibility of augmented BA care (e.g., Collaborative Assessment and Management of Suicidality [CAMS]; Jobes, 2006; referral for a medication evaluation), transition to a different type of treatment altogether, or hospitalization/residential care. More generally, a therapist might consider monitoring suicidality in the context of a BA approach, and if the adolescent does not respond to treatment, the therapist could move toward augmentation with components of other treatment modalities, or if the behavior is escalating, pursue another treatment altogether. For those with chronic suicidality there must always be an assessment of whether the adolescent would be better served by an alternative treatment such as DBT (as in the case of concomitant emotion dysregulation; see Chapter 2). The bottom line is that suicidality should not be ignored or considered a side effect of depression that will remit as the depression remits (Jobes, 2006). It must always be prioritized, adequately assessed, and addressed directly.

An example of chronic suicidality comes from Zach, the 17-year-old boy whose case was presented in Chapter 2. As noted, at the time he was seen, Zach had struggled with suicidality for the last several years, and although he had never made a suicide attempt, he talked openly about ending his life, using a range of different methods that included electrocuting himself. In the assessment, Zach endorsed thoughts of suicide weekly, and his level of suicidality became an ongoing element of discussion between Zach and his therapist. In completing a functional analysis of the behavior, Zach noted that while he had thoughts of suicide on a daily basis, they emerged more consistently in the context of disappointing interactions or experiences related to his mother, and it was during such moments, which he felt were predictable, that he actually considered carrying out a plan, such as getting into a tub full of water along with a toaster. Given Zach's chronic suicidality, Zach's therapist discussed his case in supervision on a number of occasions and considered several options over the course of his treatment. Ultimately, he was not referred to other treatment, because his suicidality was not accompanied by extreme emotion dysregulation. Likewise, hospitalization was not sought, because Zach was not deemed to be at imminent risk. Although he had struggled with suicidality for several years, he was now engaged in treatment, he openly talked about his ideation, and he had reluctantly agreed to a safety plan. Instead, Zach and his therapist focused on making suicide a target of treatment and continued to have open and transparent conversations about it, ensuring that Zach's primary caregivers (father, aunt, and uncle) had safety proofed their home and were aware of times when Zach was at greater risk. Making suicide an ongoing target of treatment involved conceptualizing it as the ultimate form of avoidance, helping Zach identify alternative coping strategies, planning for skills use following visits and interactions with his mother, and reinforcing his ongoing efforts to increase "pump you up" activities, including social connections to expand his social support network. Although Zach continued to have thoughts of suicide throughout the course of his treatment, he showed significant progress in being able to predict and manage these thoughts, with no escalation to actual suicidal or self-harming behaviors.

Family and/or Environmental Circumstances

Ongoing family circumstances can often derail therapy. They may include family conflict and stressors such as parental illness, financial hardship, and lack of parental support of the therapy process. The key to handling such issues in A-BAP really centers on working with the adolescent to understand the impact of family issues on the depression and how these issues interfere with the use of BA strategies, such as activation and goal setting, to manage depression.

Parents Who Are Not Supportive of Activation Approaches

One of the most important aspects of the A-BAP centers on successfully motivating adolescents to engage in guided activation between therapy sessions. The BA premise is that adolescents who are willing to "experiment" by taking small steps between sessions, then come back and discuss what happened with their therapist, likely make progress at a faster rate. Successfully getting an adolescent activated, however, often involves factors far beyond the adolescent's willingness to participate in experimentation. More specifically, full implementation of activation in adolescents frequently requires the support of parents and caregivers, and as such, the therapist's efforts to activate an adolescent can depend to a large degree on parents' buy-in and support of the process. Monetary and financial resources (within limits) are sometimes needed for activation, as are "permissions" to engage in appropriate activities. Over the course of developing the A-BAP approach, it was our experience that parents do not always fully appreciate their role in the activation process. Toward this end, we made significant efforts to offer parents psychoeducation with regard to the model, specifically emphasizing the important role that parents play in the activation process. Parental failure to "buy-in" to their role in supporting increased activation becomes a contextual issue that the BA therapist must manage. This issue is addressed at the onset of therapy by presenting the treatment model to both adolescents and parents, with attention to their respective roles and expectations. However, many family issues can still play a role in the treatment process. For some parents, financial concerns come into play; for others, the issues center around parenting beliefs (e.g., kids need to show responsibility and earn their own way; there is no going out until chores are completed), parental inconvenience (e.g., providing transportation to and from activities that may occur later into the evening), and/or parenting fears (e.g., refusal to allow an adolescent to attend a party if they do not know the peers' parents or to ride the bus in certain parts of town, or after a certain time in the evening). While we would never suggest that parents compromise their family values in support of A-BAP treatment, we do suggest that therapists have clear and transparent conversations with parents who are not supportive of activation approaches. The focus of such conversations centers on the role of activation in A-BAP, the importance of supporting adolescents in their efforts, and the importance of trying to negotiate with adolescents to reach a reasonable solution toward activation if what they are asking for does not fit with parenting values. And while the A-BAP therapist can offer a great deal of psychoeducation regarding the role of activation in the A-BAP treatment, the conversation must ultimately identify, validate, then problem-solve barriers the parents might be facing and address their underlying concern/fear. It can be useful for the therapist to remind parents that their son or daughter is engaging in the difficult work of trying something different, and that he or she is asking them to do the same.

An example of parental barriers to treatment comes from a 15-year-old adolescent girl we worked with named Kate. Kate attended a private school and by virtue of this choice, none of her friends lived nearby or in her neighborhood. This was very challenging for Kate, and in fact, it contributed to her feelings of depression and social isolation. As part of her activation plan, Kate wanted to meet her girlfriends in the downtown area to do some shopping on a weekend—something her friends at school frequently did. Using skills she learned as part of goal setting (Session 6: Goal Setting), Kate planned this activity very effectively. She asked her friends early in the week so as not to be disappointed in hearing that they had other plans, and talked through a plan that would allow them to meet. Because her girlfriends would be taking the bus downtown and meeting at one of their favorite stores, Kate had plans to do the same—that is, until she ran the idea by her mother. The whole idea of this plan was very frightening to Kate's mother, who ultimately said "no"—that Kate could not ride the city bus, and she could not go shopping downtown with a group of friends. Kate came back to her next session very demoralized, noting that she did everything she could to plan appropriately, only to have to go back to her friends and let them know that her mother would not allow her to go. Upon having her plans denied, Kate was unable to use her skills; instead, she did nothing. Kate continued to feel sad, lonely, and hopeless, unsure that her mother would ever allow her to engage in such an activity. In meeting with Kate's mother to provide psychoeducation about the importance of activation, it became clear that Kate's mother had very strong worries about Kate's safety if she rode the bus or hung out "downtown." More specifically, Kate's mother shared a traumatic experience she had as a young woman and her fear that Kate would have a similar traumatic experience. She specifically worried about Kate riding the bus alone, as well as the possibility of Kate getting lost and being on her own in a big city in which she had little experience. Through lots of discussion, a referral for her own therapy, negotiation, and the idea of "practicing" the activity, the therapist was able to help Kate advocate for herself and her desires, while offering Kate's mother some reassurance that Kate had the ability to handle this situation competently. In the end, Kate negotiated a plan with her mother that included her mother driving her to a friend's home so Kate and her friend could ride the bus together. Prior to this, however, Kate and her family would "practice" the activity by riding the specific bus line downtown and walking around the downtown area where Kate would be shopping with her friends, such that Kate would have some familiarity with it before doing it on her own with her friends. Although it remained anxiety provoking, Kate's mother was able to see

Kate as the competent young woman that she truly was and trust that she and her friend could safely and successfully navigate the trip.

Challenges with Managing Family Conflict

Family conflict can pose a threat to any individual treatment process with adolescents, because the therapist is often in a position of trying to negotiate with people who are not routinely in the room. In the A-BAP, we actively involve parents in the treatment, providing not only a great deal of psychoeducation about depression but also teaching communication and support skills to parents. We do this to help manage the inevitable conflict that arises for parents in response to a very irritable teen and the underappreciation they often feel as a result. In particular, as outlined in Session 2 (Situation–Activity–Mood Cycle), the psychoeducation focuses on providing support for parents and placing their adolescent's challenging behaviors in the context of depression, specifically emphasizing that this is not a willful or rejecting behavior that the adolescent can turn "on" or "off." This typically goes a long way in helping to manage conflict because parents are often able to walk away from such meetings with a new framework within which to place their teen's behavior, and one that ultimately feels less personal to them.

Another source of conflict that often arises comes from the adolescents themselves, with ongoing complaints that their parents are unreasonable and inflexible. At times the therapist may agree with this assessment. In situations in which the therapist feels that the adolescent cannot make appreciable progress without a more family-based intervention, he or she may first attempt to augment the BA therapy with more family sessions in which BA strategies can be taught to parents and used to problem-solve conflict. If this is not successful and significant conflict continues, a referral for more intensive family therapy or a treatment referral for the parent may be in order.

Summary

Previously we outlined some of the more common treatment challenges related to working with depressed adolescents. As noted early on, these challenges are viewed as a routine part of working with adolescents and their families. With all, the therapist is strongly encouraged to fully utilize the tools that the BA approach has to offer, particularly the use of functional analysis in understanding each challenge and outlining the best course of action. Prioritizing issues as treatment targets and considering them in the context of "avoidance behaviors" are of utmost importance. While the therapist is encouraged to manage treatment challenges in the context of BA therapy by helping the adolescent utilize applicable skills, augmentation with other approaches is sometimes needed. In the event that the challenge cannot be adequately managed or if symptoms escalate, the therapist must always evaluate the potential need for other interventions. We think, however, that this is generally not necessary and that most treatment challenges can be managed adequately within the context of the A-BAP approach.

CHAPTER 5

Applications of Behavioral Activation with Other Clinical Samples/Situations

The A-BAP was created to treat youth with depression; based on our work to date, however, we believe that the A-BAP, or components of the A-BAP approach, may be useful in working with youth with other mental health problems, as well as preventive work with youth with medical issues and/or lifestyle challenges. Given its idiographic and modular nature, the A-BAP is well-suited for application to other problems and populations, including generalized or social anxiety, mild disruptive behavior, and chronic illness and weight management problems, although it has not yet been formally tested with these populations. When extending the A-BAP to other populations, therapists are encouraged to maintain "flexibility within fidelity" (Kendall & Beidas, 2007) by carefully balancing adherence to A-BAP principles, with efforts to individualize. Pragmatically, therapists should utilize clinical judgment, consultation with colleagues, the existing evidence base, and supervision to make changes and extensions appropriately. In Chapter 2, we discussed youth for whom the A-BAP may not be sufficient, including but not limited to youth who present with extreme emotion regulation problems, chronic and severe suicidality/self-injurious behaviors, and psychosis. In this chapter, we focus on populations for whom modification of the A-BAP approach may be reasonable, and we provide some guidance about how to modify it appropriately for adolescents with generalized or social anxiety, mild disruptive behavior, chronic illness, weight management problems and other extensions. Case examples are included to help illustrate such modifications.

Youth with Other Psychopathology

Based on our work to date, we believe that adolescents who present with anxiety or mild to moderate disruptive behavior without comorbid depression are likely good candidates for the A-BAP. Some important exceptions include youth with panic disorder, obsessive–compulsive disorder (OCD), or severe posttraumatic stress disorder (PTSD), who would be better served by interventions specifically designed and proven efficacious for these problems. However, adolescents who have an anxious temperament and present with mild to moderate social phobia or generalized anxiety disorder (GAD) would likely benefit from the A-BAP. Additionally, adolescents with a trauma history who have undergone successful treatment for acute trauma and present with residual depression may also be good candidates for the A-BAP. As discussed earlier, adolescents with ADHD and mild oppositional defiant disorder (ODD) are good candidates; however, if youth have severe ODD, conduct disorder, or severe substance abuse problems, the A-BAP may not be a good fit. Components of the BA approach (e.g., activity scheduling) may, however, be useful strategies to include in treatment, especially as these youth work to develop more prosocial behavioral and friendship patterns.

Anxiety

Given the significant co-occurrence of depression and anxiety in adolescence (Garber & Weersing, 2010), it is quite common for adolescents to present with symptoms from both domains. Initial trials of the A-BAP were administered to adolescents with a primary depressive disorder (McCauley et al., 2015), but during our initial trial, we found the A-BAP to be effective for comorbid anxiety. Early work with adults receiving a BA treatment for worry (Chen, Liu, Rapee, & Pillay, 2013) has been promising and adds more support for using a similar approach with adolescents. In turn, even in the absence of a depressive disorder, we support extending the A-BAP for use with adolescents with a primary anxiety disorder. Consistent with treatments specifically designed for anxiety, therapists using the A-BAP approach should pay close attention to understanding and integrating the adolescent's symptoms of anxiety in the initial formulation and model. For example, instead of depression, the primary treatment target may be worry or fear of social situations, which would easily fit with the BA model of loss of reinforcing experiences and secondary problems (e.g., avoidance) that maintain the anxiety. Given that many times anxiety disorders represent the intensification of a normal personality disposition to worry and heightened reactivity to one's environment (Akiskal, 2007), when anxiety is a primary target, consideration of temperament is important. When generating the initial formulation and model, the therapist should also take care to explore how the adolescent's temperament affects his or her life circumstances; emotional responses; actions; and, in turn, the secondary consequences. A related issue is that therapists should be attuned to the anxious adolescent's potential experience of in-session anxiety when meeting a new person and disclosing personal information. Therapists can easily adapt the A-BAP approach to support adolescents by enlisting more parental involvement, teaching basic relaxation skills at the beginning of treatment rather than waiting until Session 5 (Problem Solving), and expanding psychoeducation to include information about anxiety, in addition to depression. Maintaining a focus on the adolescent's particular target symptom will continue to be important as the therapist transitions to monitoring situation–activity–mood and could result in coaching the adolescent to monitor situation–worry–activity. A-BAP's explicit focus on overcoming avoidance is easily applicable to anxiety and compatible with evidence-based treatment for anxiety. Therapists will find that using the goal-setting framework, including scheduling mini-steps and anticipating barriers, functions in a similar manner as developing a fear hierarchy and working through an exposure protocol. Whenever an exposure-based intervention is utilized, it is critical to educate the adolescent and his or her parents about the importance of riding out the anxiety when engaging in the exposure exercise. Failure to do this can result in the avoidance or escape behavior being reinforced and likely strengthened, rather than achieving the treatment goal of the adolescent experiencing reward or reinforcement as a result of staying in the anxiety-provoking situation.

Vignette 1

Claire was an introverted 15-year-old girl who presented with social anxiety, somatic complaints, and irritability. She did not have friends to speak of, and her peer relationships were limited to highly structured interactions, such as in-class groupwork. Claire had always been shy and inclined to spend time with just one or two friends rather than with large groups. During early sessions, when determining how the A-BAP model worked for her, it became clear that, over time, as she moved from childhood to adolescence, her parents' scaffolding of her social activities decreased, which led to decreased involvement in social activities, low confidence about how to interact with peers, and high levels of social anxiety and loneliness. The prospect of being put in a social situation prompted Claire to experience high levels of anxiety, sadness, and irritability. Not surprisingly, she frequently avoided social situations, which resulted in Claire feeling lonely and hopeless about ever having a close relationship, including friendships and romantic relationships. In the first part of treatment, the therapist provided psychoeducation to Claire and her parents that focused on anxiety, including the importance of approaching feared situations in conjunction with aversive activities. The therapist brought forward the content of Session 8, "Overcoming Avoidance," supplemented it with information about anxiety and integrated it with the psychoeducation on depression in Session 2. When focusing on interconnections among situations, worry, mood, and activities (from Session 2), it also became clear that decreasing Claire's anxiety, bolstering her social skills, and improving her comfort in social situations were key to improving her life. Claire's therapist worked to teach her relaxation strategies early on in order to help set the stage for trying social experiments. Specifically, instead of waiting until Session 5 (Problem Solving), the therapist introduced some relaxation skills in the second session. In Session 3, when discussing getting active and learning how to engage in goal-directed rather than mood-directed behavior, Claire and her therapist discussed how her social anxiety was driving her behavior and, in turn, they started to discuss how she might begin to act according to a plan rather than according to her "gut." This also was reviewed when evaluating the short- and long-term consequences of her behavior in Session 4. The therapist and Claire went through examples of responding in ways to immediately ease her anxiety about events (i.e., turning down an invitation to the Homecoming Dance) that had negative, long-term consequences (feeling lonely and left out when looking at her friends' Homecoming pictures on social media). When learning about goal setting in Session 6, Claire knew she wanted to feel more comfortable in social situations and do more things with friends, but she felt overwhelmed and unsure about where to start. Claire's therapist emphasized that they could take things slowly and that once she began to practice goal-setting, she would likely be able to generalize the framework to more and more situations and goals. In the process of identifying and mapping out Claire's first "SMART" goal, she and her therapist used multiple BA approaches that were also consistent with common anxiety interventions that focus on fear hierarchies. Specifically, she and her therapist used COPE (from Session 5) as a method to brainstorm—Claire first engaged in relaxation to calm down. Her therapist asked her to rate her anxiety on a 1 to 10 scale, and when she was at a "2" or lower, they would take the next step, which was to identify all of the possible options. During this process, the therapist frequently asked Claire to rate her anxiety, and anytime she was above a "2" (due to the anxiety triggered by talking about possible future activities and behaviors), Claire was coached to engage in relaxation strategies. As the conversation about various options for SMART goals proceeded, despite exploration of increasingly difficult strategies, she was able to keep her anxiety at a low level. Claire and her therapist rated the options according to how anxiety provoking each would be, which led them to select and sequence the various options.

For her first SMART goal, on the following Wednesday, Claire planned to ask a particular peer in her youth group if she wanted to go to a movie that weekend. This peer was someone Claire often sat by and with whom she already felt comfortable, but they had never spent time outside of youth group or church. Claire completed Handout 23 ("Goal Setting" worksheet), including outlining mini-steps of (1) scheduling time to research reasonable movie options online prior to meeting with the youth group and to identify two or three PG- or PG-13-rated movies in town; (2) scheduling time to practice her planned approach in front of a mirror and with her mother prior to the youth group meeting (this included a couple of opening questions about her weekend plan and whether she had seen the selected movie options); (3) clarifying her plan to go to the meeting early to decrease potential anxiety about being late; (4) making a plan for Claire try to sit by the peer, with the backup plan of finding her during the bathroom break if they did not end up sitting together; and (5) scheduling next steps, if in fact the peer could go to the movie, including exchanging phone numbers and determining when and how they would communicate about a final plan. Then, Claire and her therapist engaged in a role play in order to practice how Claire would initiate the conversation. For the last 10 minutes of the session, Claire's mother joined them, so that Claire could share her SMART goal and mini-steps, and also so Claire could inquire about ways she was hoping her mother could support her and confirm the times they could do this (i.e., engaging in a role play of what Claire was going to say to her peer; making sure she could get to the youth group early this week; confirming timing options for the weekend movie with regard to her parents' availability to take her, or possibly both of them, to the movie). With Claire's mother present, they collaboratively anticipated potential barriers to Claire's mini-steps, such as getting in a traffic jam on the way to the meeting and being later than Claire would like, the peer not being at the youth group this week, and the possibility that the conversation might go differently than expected. The therapist emphasized that even with thorough planning and solid effort, real life is hard to plan, but learning how to be flexible and able to cope with changes in plans is both a part of the process and yields important data about how to move forward with Claire's goal, and that because this was an experiment, any outcome would be helpful. While early on it was important for Claire to feel calm and relaxed prior to engaging in problem solving, as treatment progressed, Claire eventually began to practice coping effectively even when feeling anxious.

Disruptive Behavior

Despite the high frequency of comorbid depression and disruptive behavior symptoms (Angold, Costello, & Erkanli, 1999), integrated treatments that target these co-occurring disorders have mostly been tested in children and adolescents up through age 13 (Wolff & Ollendick, 2006; Weisz et al., 2012). During our initial trial, we found the A-BAP to be effective for youth with mild to moderate disruptive behavior problems. Adolescents and their parents frequently seek treatment when the teen is experiencing marked irritability or anger outbursts, as well as problems with attention. After careful assessment to rule out the presence of conduct disorder, which would indicate referral to multisystemic therapy (MST; Henggeler, Schoenwald, Borduin, Rowland, & Cunningham, 1998) or another intensive behavioral treatment involving both youth and parents, adolescents who present with anger, irritability, or oppositionality may benefit from the A-BAP. Understanding what is important to each adolescent, analyzing how existing activity choices may bring short-term payoff but carry a longer-term price, and identifying alternative appealing activities may be useful.

In the A-BAP, anger or "bursting" is conceptualized as a form of avoidance. Individuals, who, when stressed or upset, become argumentative or verbally aggressive are essentially disengaging from the person or situation rather than engaging in active problem solving. Like avoidance patterns that are characteristic of being sad or anxious, this type of behavioral pattern can also serve to precipitate or exacerbate a downward spiral due to the consequences of family, friends, coaches, and teachers distancing themselves, or result in loss of privileges (e.g., being grounded). Engaging adolescents in situation–activity–mood monitoring to learn about the antecedents and consequences of "bursting" is a helpful way to improve insight about how actions affect others and, in turn, negatively affect the adolescent's own life. Once again, it is important to use words that resonate with the adolescent, so you may ask the adolescent to pay attention to situation–anger–activity. Youth with attention problems and disruptive behavior often benefit from learning and practicing problem-solving skills given their reactivity and impulsivity. The A-BAP problem-solving framework (COPE) teaches the adolescent skills to use when he or she faces a challenge or makes a decision or does something that leads to a negative consequence. Supporting the adolescent to develop the habit of calming, considering all options, and selecting and evaluating a choice is typically very helpful. Since disruptive behavior is better targeted by preventing it rather than managing it in the moment, it is typically more fruitful to invest one's efforts in teaching prevention skills and clarifying the context that sets the stage for disruptive behavior, such as being around a certain peer or caregiver, being in a specific setting (e.g., school) or with family at home or in a specific state (e.g., being hungry or not getting enough sleep). It is also helpful to focus on identifying and practicing ways the adolescent can cope in order to deescalate appropriately by taking a break or engaging in deep breathing. Another angle is to teach the adolescent to self-reward when he or she has successes, in addition to supporting parents' efforts to attend to the positive and not just the negative behaviors that often grab attention by encouraging them to highlight and reward positive behavior or the absence of aversive behavior. Therapists should also consider including parent-training techniques such as how to best respond to disruptive behaviors. Additionally, engaging in rewarding, healthy, and pleasant activities is incompatible with anger. In turn, a helpful preventive strategy is to schedule one's life with a steady dose of "pump you up" activities, in balance with mastery and developmentally required activities (e.g., school) in order to decrease the opportunity to become angry.

Vignette 2

Jake, a 14-year-old boy, had a long history of problems with attention and oppositionality. From kindergarten to the beginning of middle school, with the support of ADHD medication, Jake demonstrated gains with regard to concentration and hyperactivity. However, upon starting middle school, he began to struggle with increasingly impairing irritability, disrespectful and mean behavior, and defiance and oppositionality, which prompted his parents to bring him in for treatment. Initial work focused on identifying his target symptoms, which included antagonizing his sister, talking back to his parents and teachers, and often refusing to get off his game system to do homework. Using functional analysis, the therapist generated a model of Jake's problem behavior, which demonstrated that certain contexts (e.g., having idle time at school, at home, or in the car) led to him feeling irritated, bored, and restless, which, in turn, led him to tease his sister, play his video games regardless of whether he was supposed to, and often make what he thought were funny, disrespectful comments to his family, his teachers, and peers. Secondary consequences of his actions included frequently being grounded and sent to detention; often being in conflict with his family; and losing the privilege of using his phone, his laptop and game system; as well as having very few close relationships. Jake was insistent that others caused all of his problems because they were too demanding or too annoying. In the first session, Jake's therapist outlined the model of behavior and change and was careful to avoid getting into a debate about who was at fault. Through detailing how they would engage in "Test It Out" activities designed to make his life better through increased access to his games and improved friendships, Jake was gradually responsive to trying new things and understood that they could not do too much about others' behavior. The next steps (Session 2) involved examining patterns between his situation and context, his behavior and activity, and his mood, which revealed that boredom or confusion was frequently paired with Jake's acting out and getting in trouble or being disrespectful to others. This process highlighted that although, in the short-term, acting out was effective in regard to decreasing boredom and possibly getting others to laugh, the long-term "price" was loss of privileges and often ongoing confusion due to difficulty paying attention in class or completing homework or chores. In essence, Jake avoided feeling stupid or confused by being a class clown. Jake and his therapist worked together to identify typical triggers (e.g., classes he found challenging; feeling jealous of his sister's successes) and responses (e.g., anger, irritation, boredom, confusion, feeling stupid, or desiring attention from peers), as well as his avoidance patterns (e.g., disrupting the class by talking to a friend, making a joke or interrupting the teacher, insulting his sister, ignoring his parents' commands), in order that Jake might begin to engage in alternative coping (e.g., asking a question in class, getting help from his tutor or a friend, communicating with his parents about the difficulty of having a "perfect" sister). As a result, over time, he was open to including his parents and even certain teachers in helping him to be aware of TRAP-TRAC patterns, which gradually decreased his target behaviors and increased his opportunity to engage in "pump you up" activities given that he was no longer grounded.

Youth with Medical Problems

In addition to youth presenting with select psychopathology, we also see the A-BAP as a useful intervention for youth with other presentations, including chronic illness, pain, and weight management problems. Certainly some adolescents facing these challenges may also demonstrate clinical depression, but we see a role for BA even in the absence of a depressive disorder and describe two such applications below.

Chronic Illness

Youth with chronic illness are more likely than peers to have a set of challenges or limitations in their daily lives that puts them at risk of poor psychosocial outcomes (Law et al., 2006; Maslow, Haydon, McRee, Ford, & Halpern, 2011; Stam, Hartman, Deurloo, Groothoff, & Grootenhuis, 2006). Relatedly, the BA model of depression posits that a life that is not sufficiently rewarding is considered to be a proximal risk factor for depression (Martell et al., 2001) and has been pilot tested with adults with cancer (Ryba, Lejuez, & Hopko, 2014). The A-BAP can be a useful intervention to enrich daily lives and prevent the onset or worsening of depression. Modifications and considerations include using terminology that fits the patient. For example, in lieu of *depression,* the adolescent may conceptualize the root of his or her challenges to be his or her illness (e.g., pain, Crohn's disease) or have his or her own word for the most challenging symptoms (e.g., "feeling blah"). It is important to validate that the illness has and will continue to be a part of the adolescent's life, and that proactively filling his or her life with opportunities for pleasure, joy, and mastery, and overcoming any avoidance patterns will prevent the occurrence of downward spirals. In working with an adolescent with chronic medical symptoms, it is important to engage in thorough situation–activity–mood monitoring in order to understand how he or she responds to symptoms. The adolescent is likely an expert in regard to living with chronic illness.

When working with youth with chronic illness, it may be helpful for therapists to modify their expectations about frequency of sessions or about their cancellation policies. It is not unusual for adolescents with chronic illnesses to have worsening symptoms that occur suddenly and may interfere with their ability to attend a session. Keeping them to a "24-hour" cancellation policy may financially punish adolescents or their families for unavoidable, last-minute cancellations. When adolescents have great difficulty coming into the office for a session because of illness, it is a reasonable idea to decrease the frequency of face-to-face sessions and plan some sort of check-in over the telephone or through some other confidential technological means.

Vignette 3

A-BAP was used successfully for Maya, a 12-year-old girl, to help her deal with chronic knee pain, which led to school avoidance and social isolation, and eventually resulted in mild depression. Prior to presenting to the A-BAP therapist, Maya had engaged in a brief course of CBT for pain that had in many ways given her a great set of skills, including imagery and relaxation, and had taken a comprehensive psychoeducation course on pain and how to cope. However, she had difficulty using the skills on a daily basis and had developed the behavioral pattern of refusing to go to school due to pain. This set her up to fall behind with academics, as well as become socially isolated, which made going to school less reinforcing and more difficult to do. Her situation–activity–mood charts revealed that her natural response to pain, to stay home in bed, had the short-term effect of making her feel good but the negative long-term consequences of bringing her down due to her stress about schoolwork and attendance, as well as feeling out of the loop with friends. Using the A-BAP principles of engaging in goal-directed behavior (Session 2) and using TRAP-TRAC to identify and modify avoidance patterns (Session 8), Maya worked with her therapist to develop a plan to get her out of her current TRAP (Trigger: pain; Response: fatigue, anergia; Avoidance Pattern: refusing to go to school) and get her back on TRAC (Trigger: pain; Response: fatigue, anergia; Alternative Coping: go to school). When Maya faced pain, her natural, understandable response was to feel fatigued and unenergetic. She learned to view this response as a sign to engage in goal-directed behavior (go to school) instead of mood- or pain-directed behavior (stay in bed). Ongoing mood monitoring revealed that when she was able to go to school, Maya enjoyed the long-term consequences of improved mood as a result of staying on top of schoolwork and feeling connected with friends. Maya's pain was somewhat constant, but she learned how to minimize its negative impact on her life as a whole.

Weight Management

Youth with weight management problems are also good candidates for BA. For this population, the A-BAP is best considered to be a component of a multidisciplinary program of care given the importance of focused, professional support, with nutrition, physical activity, and attention to the complex environmental factors that can contribute to weight gain. Recent work suggests that depressed adult women who received a behavioral weight loss treatment utilizing BA principles demonstrated greater improvement in depression than did women receiving a weight loss treatment alone; of note, the women whose depression decreased lost significantly more weight (Busch et al., 2013; Pagoto, Bodenlos, Schneider,

Olendzki, & Spates, 2008). As with other extensions of the A-BAP, it is important to use language that resonates with the adolescent when describing the target behavior or treatment goal. Clarification of terms and goals is the first step in determining how BA works for adolescents. The therapist and adolescent then co-construct the BA model by identifying the contextual factors and life circumstances that lead to the negative emotions, which in turn foster activities that interfere with effective weight management. The therapist should be curious about the role of nutrition and physical activity for the adolescent in order to understand how situations, moods, and actions interrelate. Involving parents is particularly important with weight management given the prominent role of the home with regard to food and nutrition, family meals, and parent modeling and facilitation of activity.

Vignette 4

Alex, a 15-year-old boy, found that the A-BAP helped him with his goal of losing weight. Throughout his life, he had tried numerous strategies to lose weight; however, despite some short-term improvement, he was unable to find anything that worked consistently, and over time his weight continued to climb. In the first session, when creating his A-BAP model, time was spent discussing his early childhood history given its impact on his current life circumstances. Specifically, he described a long history of being bullied and teased by peers initially due to his awkwardness and social skill deficits and, over time, due to being overweight. Additionally, he described his home life to be somewhat isolative due to having "homebody" parents with whom he spent the majority of his free time. As he moved into adolescence, Alex had more interest in spending time outside of the home and connecting with peers; however, he did not feel confident or skilled in these domains and lived an isolated, sedentary lifestyle. Alex and his therapist determined that in addition to being overweight, his life circumstances led to feeling sad and embarrassed, as well as angry at his parents. His response to these feelings, though, was to ruminate about his predicament, be argumentative with his parents, and spend his time at home online or playing video games. Because of his resentment and frustration, Alex initially refused to involve his parents in therapy sessions. Instead of pushing this issue, his therapist proceeded with the A-BAP protocol in order to build Alex's skills set, including an emphasis on goal setting (Session 6) and identification of barriers (Session 7). Alex readily learned the skills and created effective goals to increase his social and extra-curricular activities; however, he encountered lots of roadblocks when trying to implement his action plans. For example, Alex initially set what seemed like a SMART goal of joining a gym where an acquaintance from school was a member. Mini-steps for this goal included mapping out a public transportation route to get to the gym and scheduling a tour of the gym in order to initiate a free trial membership. Due to his insistence on keeping his parents out of this process, Alex had not communicated with them about this goal or the mini-steps until he was getting ready to leave to catch the bus to go to his scheduled tour and announced that he was going out and would be back in a couple of hours. His mother asked where he was going, which was irritating to Alex, who insisted that it was none of her business. In the absence of any context, as well as due to frustration about

Alex's poor communication and concern about him taking public transportation on his own, she told Alex that he was not allowed to take the bus alone; furthermore, he was not allowed to leave the house unless he could provide more specific information about his plans. At his next therapy session, Alex was very angry about what he saw as his mother's efforts to control him and not let him grow up. Evaluation of the internal and external barriers and ongoing experimentation with different tacks revealed that Alex's refusal to involve his parents made accomplishing many of the steps nearly impossible—he needed their help, or at least their permission and agreement, to tackle problems with transportation and family rules about social plans. After trying alternative ways around this issue with limited success, Alex agreed to try to include his parents in sessions. Through parent–adolescent sessions, Alex's parents learned that their mood-directed behavior of protecting their son from further distress from peers had contributed to his weight gain and loneliness. Alex learned that his parents needed to see him gradually demonstrate improved judgment and more effective social skills in order to feel comfortable with giving him more freedom to do things on his own and with new peers. Eventually, as Alex demonstrated successes with mini-steps toward his goals (e.g., getting his parents the names and contact information of peers' parents, going on a practice bus ride to the mall with his parents), his parents gradually became more willing to let Alex try new things and spend time with peers, and they were able to offer instrumental support that Alex increasingly was open to accept, such as providing rides and being open to having his friends come to the house. By the end of treatment, Alex had not only improved his relationship with his parents and begun to develop friendships with same-age peers, he had also gradually begun to lose weight. The A-BAP component set the stage for Alex and his parents to initiate work with a nutritionist and a fitness coach with success.

Other Extensions

The A-BAP is a good match for less cognitively mature youth who may struggle with effectively learning and applying cognitive interventions, as well as for youth who do not present with prominent negative cognitions. Focused work on A-BAP strategies is typically doable for even young adolescents, even if they do not have a lot of insight about why they are experiencing depression. As with all interventions for young or cognitively immature individuals, involving parents with treatment can facilitate the uptake of skills, as well as provide the therapist with sufficient information about the child's context and history.

Vignette 5

Nina, a 15-year-old young woman with cognitive delay, had become depressed in the context of starting high school. Initially, Nina did not resonate with the concept of depression and was insistent that high school simply "sucked" and there was nothing to be done about it. She was willing to try therapy and also to include her mother in sessions. Constructing her BA model of depression revealed that Nina was often confused and/or overwhelmed by the social milieu that was much bigger than her junior high and complicated by peers engaging in more mature and high-risk behavior, including smoking pot, using over-the-counter drugs, and engaging in public displays of affection. Nina frequently felt lonely and sad, which in turn resulted in her withdrawal and avoidance of peers. Nina was very open to engaging in BA and, with the help of her therapist and her mother, was able to learn how therapy skills could help her to make sense of high school and all of its challenges. For example, early on, given Nina's frequent feelings of confusion and being overwhelmed, her therapist taught her the COPE problem-solving framework (typically introduced in Session 5, but was introduced to Nina in Session 2 given its importance to help her manage her emotions). Nina resonated with the clear, stepwise process and readily learned the steps, which she found to be quite helpful. Specifically, she learned that when she felt frustrated or upset, she would first try to get calm and to clarify the problem (e.g., being around classmates who were high and trying to get her to use pot), identify options (e.g., ignore them, use humor to distract them, be assertive, get help from others), pick and perform an option, and evaluate. After some trial and error, Nina engaged in role plays with her therapist in order to get practice with language and tone that were effective with peers. When faced with a challenge, something she frequently encountered, Nina finally had a concrete way to approach it, as well as clear helpers when she struggled to fit her challenges to the steps (i.e., initially, her therapist but eventually her mother as well). Over time, she was able to use her COPE skills independently and without prompting from others, which also set the stage for her to engage in goal setting and modifying avoidance patterns.

Summary

Many of the important considerations that are true for using the A-BAP for youth with depression are also critical for youth struggling with other types of symptoms or challenges that commonly co-occur with depression. Therapists are advised to use the language that resonates with the adolescent when initiating treatment. The term may be *depression*, but it could also be *anxiety, anger, pain,* or *"the blahs."* It also is critical to measure important symptoms on a regular basis. This can be accomplished by adding an appropriate measure, such as a self-report form of anxiety or disruptive behavior or improvising by adding items to the depression scale (e.g., to measure pain or gastrointestinal distress). As the evidence base for the A-BAP grows, we anticipate that it will continue to be applied as a stand-alone treatment, and that some therapists will utilize individual modules for a broad range of disorders in youth, including depression, comorbid psychopathology, and medical and health conditions.

A-BAP Treatment Sessions

MODULE 1
Getting Started

SESSION 1

Introduction to the Adolescent Behavioral Activation Program (A-BAP)

Suggested Total Session Time: 45–50 minutes

Session Overview

Goals

Session 1 focuses on building rapport and introducing the structure for this individualized treatment. There are three main goals in this session:

1. Review the structure of therapy.
2. Review history with both the adolescent and the parent(s) for integration into a functional analytic framework and the BA model.
3. Introduce the BA model of depression and treatment, integrating psychoeducation about depression.

Structure and Teaching Points

Session 1 is structured to include both the adolescent and parent(s), followed by a brief check-in with the adolescent. After reviewing the structure of treatment within the BA model, the focus is on outlining the connection between the adolescent's life events, daily hassles, current problems, and symptoms, and the way the adolescent has tried to cope. The main teaching points are as follows:

- Life events/daily hassles can lead to feeling sad and fatigued, as well as having low energy and a generally negative mood.
- These symptoms are sometimes labeled as "depression."

- There is a natural response to these feelings—people do things to make these feelings go away and attempt to cope.
- Discuss what the adolescent has done to feel better (e.g., avoid school, friends, and activities).
- Highlight those behaviors that make depression worse rather than better and how these behaviors can become secondary problems, creating a "vicious cycle."
- Point out that BA seeks to break the "vicious cycle" of depression by focusing on and addressing the secondary problems.
- The end result is to help adolescents ***get back on track and feel better.***

Session Agenda

Adolescent and Parent(s) Together

- Check-In
- Key Concepts for today's session:
  - Concept 1: Structure of Therapy
  - Concept 2: BA Model
    - Handout 1 (Teaching Guide): "Behavioral Activation Model"
    - Handout 2 (Worksheet): "How Behavioral Activation Works for You"

Adolescent Only

- Complete the SMFQ/PHQ-9.
- Setting the Agenda:
  - What we will cover today
  - Adolescent's Agenda
- Key Concepts for today's session:
  - Concept 3: Activity Monitoring
- "Test It Out" activity for the week: Handout 3 (Test It Out): "Activity Monitoring"

Materials You Need to Have Ready

- Today's Agenda
- Setting-related paperwork (e.g., release of information [ROI], consent for care, if indicated)
- SMFQ/PHQ-9
- Handout 1: "Behavioral Activation Model" (two copies)
- Handout 2: "How Behavioral Activation Works for You" (two copies)
- Handout 3: "Activity Monitoring"

Outline of Session

ADOLESCENT AND PARENT(S) TOGETHER

Check-In

- Welcome the adolescent and parent(s) to the session.
- Share how much you look forward to working together.

Review Today's Agenda

Review Today's Agenda, highlighting that today will not be a typical session, going over a few business items, and spending most of the session with adolescent and parent(s) together. At the end of the session, we will spend some time with the adolescent alone.

Key Concepts for Today's Session

"The goal today is to spend the majority of the session talking about the structure of therapy and how the behavioral activation model fits for you. We will end the session by spending some time with you individually."

Concept 1: Review the Structure of Treatment

"In getting started, let's talk a bit about the structure of the A-BAP treatment. In the A-BAP, there are three major roles. The A-BAP uses a coaching model. You will be the primary player; I am here to support and coach you, and we will ask your parent(s) to also support your efforts. This treatment is typically a short-term treatment that lasts about 12 or so sessions. Most sessions will be about 45–50 minutes."

Review the basic structure of BA treatment sessions.

Roles in the A-BAP Treatment

- Adolescent—primary player
- Therapist—coach
- Parent(s)—support person(s)

Format of Sessions

- Most sessions will follow the same format. Typically, we start by meeting individually with the adolescent for about 25–30 minutes, followed by a brief family meeting or individual time with the parent(s) for 15–20 minutes.
- We will always work from an agenda and always start by completing a short questionnaire (e.g., the SMFQ or PHQ-9), that will help us understand symptoms the adolescent may be experiencing.

- Sessions involve learning a variety of strategies to better understand and cope with depression.
- There will be regular "check-ins" regarding possible emergent issues (e.g., significant stressors and thoughts of suicide) at each session with interventions as needed (confidentiality limits, etc.).
- "Test It Out" activities: Viewed as an important part of the treatment process for both the adolescent and parent(s).
  - The focus will be on learning key elements reviewed in session.
  - Represents opportunities to practice new skills and turn them into healthy habits.
  - Are designed to minimize time burden for completion.

Concept 2: Introduction of the BA Model

"Now that we have talked a little about the structure of therapy, I would like us to talk about the behavioral activation model and how it fits your life and experiences."

Introduce Handout 1 (Teaching Guide): "Behavioral Activation Model"

Using Handout 1 (Teaching Guide): "Behavioral Activation Model," present a general example of the model to the adolescent. The main teaching points are as follows:

- Life events/daily hassles can lead to feeling sad and fatigued, as well as having low energy and a generally negative mood.
- These symptoms are sometimes labeled as "depression."
- There is a natural response to these feelings—people do things to make these feelings go away and attempt to cope.
- Discuss what the adolescent has done to feel better (e.g., avoid school, friends, and activities).
- Highlight behaviors that make depression worse rather than better, and how these behaviors can become secondary problems, creating a "vicious cycle."
- Point out that BA seeks to break the "vicious cycle" of depression by focusing on and addressing the secondary problems.
- The end result is to help adolescents **get back on track and feel better.**

Introduce Handout 2 (Worksheet): "How Behavioral Activation Works for You"

- After taking the adolescent and parent(s) through the overall model, walk them through Handout 2 (Worksheet): "How Behavioral Activation Works for You," encouraging them to draw on the adolescent's and family's current situation and having them think through how the model fits.
- Make sure this is collaborative.
- Get everyone's input and approval.

- Enlist adolescent and parent(s) in making corrections, additions, and so forth.
- Highlight that you will modify details and add to the model as you become better acquainted.
- Thank the adolescent and parent(s) for giving you so much information; highlight how this information will be helpful in terms of thinking about a treatment plan.

Closing

"We have covered a lot today—and now I would like to spend some time alone with your son/daughter to begin talking about how to begin to use this model in his/her daily life."

ADOLESCENT ONLY

Complete the SMFQ/PHQ-9

"We will start each session by having you complete a questionnaire. This will give us a quick indication of how you have been feeling since we last got together, and will help us identify problems or difficulties to work on, such as difficulties with sleep or thoughts of harming yourself. This will also let us track how your feelings are changing over time."

- Ask the adolescent to complete the SMFQ or PHQ-9.
- Inform the adolescent that every week you will use the SMFQ/PHQ-9 as a guide for both of you to determine what, if anything, needs attention or should be added to the agenda.

Adolescent's Agenda

"Each time we meet, we will set an agenda. It will highlight what we cover today, and you will have an opportunity to add any items you want to make sure we talk about and discuss."

- What we will cover today
- Adolescent's Agenda
  - Particularly in Session 1, your time with the adolescent will be limited, making it hard to address his or her agenda items. You will need to structure your time such that you can cover Concept 3 and introduce the "Test It Out" activity, so you may need to carry over his or her agenda items to the next session.

Concept 3: Activity Monitoring

"Today we want to have you start paying attention to what you do and the activities in your life. When you come back next time, we will begin to look at how the activities you

choose and how what you do can affect how you feel. For example, I try to run every Saturday morning. When I do it, I feel good and have good energy. When I give in to the urge to stay in my pajamas and sit on the couch, I tend to have less energy and feel more grouchy."

"Test It Out" for the Coming Week: Introduce Handout 3 (Test It Out): "Activity Monitoring"

"As a first step, we just want to get a good sense of what you do and how you spend your time. This worksheet highlights 2 days out of each week. Let's go through what you have done today and then have you track one day on your own."

- Walk the adolescent through each hour of today, writing down what he or she did, regardless of how mundane it might seem to him or her (e.g., eating breakfast, sleeping, watching TV, driving to therapy).
- Once you have completed this example, ask the adolescent to keep on tracking the rest of today and additionally track one other day prior to his or her next appointment. Encourage him or her to bring the activity chart back, so that you can review it together.

Thanks and Next Steps

- Thank the adolescent for his or her good work and attention. Ask if there is anything that we should briefly check-in about regarding the session.
- Preview that in the next session we will start to examine the connection between what the adolescent does and how he or she feels.

SESSION 2

Situation–Activity–Mood Cycle

Suggested Total Session Time: 50–60 minutes

Session Overview

Goals

Module 1 centers on getting A-BAP started. Session 2 focuses on helping the adolescent begin to make connections between situations he or she faces, how the adolescent responds, what he or she does, and how he or she feels. There are three main goals in this session:

1. Gain a better understanding of the adolescent's relationships and activities.
2. Expand the adolescent's understanding of the relation between activity and mood.
3. Introduce the notion of "downward" and "upward" spirals, focusing particularly on the connection among situation, activity, and mood.

Structure and Teaching Points

This session is structured to include a working session with the adolescent followed by a brief check-in and teaching exercise with the parent(s). The session begins with the routine "Check-In" components (greeting, monitoring, agenda review, and homework review). The main teaching points are as follows:

- In addition to events in our environment, relationships/activities impact our mood.
- It is important to notice the connections between situations, our responses, what we do (activity), and how we feel (mood).

- Our actions can maintain, improve, or worsen our mood.
- We can get into a "downward spiral" when we react to a situation by doing something that brings down our mood and/or worsens the original problem.
- We can get into an "upward spiral" when we react to a situation by doing something that improves our mood and leads to more effective coping.
- Once you can recognize the pattern of the spiral that you are in, we will begin to teach you how to use activity to change your mood.
- With the parent(s), present and review psychoeducation related to depression.

Session Agenda

Adolescent Only

- Check-In
- Review "Test It Out": Handout 3 (Test It Out): "Activity Monitoring"
- Key Concepts for today's session:
  - Concept 1: How Relationships and Activities Impact Mood
    - Handout 4 (Worksheet): "Who and What Is on 'First' in Your Life?"
  - Concept 2: Situation–Activity–Mood Cycle
    - Handout 5 (Test It Out): Downward Spiral, Upward Spiral
- "Test It Out" activity for the week: Handout 5 (Test It Out): "Downward Spiral, Upward Spiral"

Parent(s) Only

- Key Concepts for today's session:
  - Concept 1: Depression in Adolescence
    - Handout 6 (Teaching Guide): "A Parent Guide to Adolescent Depression"
  - Concept 2: Supporting Your Adolescent Through His or Her Depression

Materials You Need to Have Ready

- Today's Agenda
- SMFQ/PHQ-9
- Handout 3 (Test It Out): "Activity Monitoring"
- Handout 4 (Worksheet): "Who and What Is on 'First' in Your Life?"
- Handout 5 (Test It Out): "Downward Spiral, Upward Spiral" (2 copies)
- Handout 6 (Teaching Guide): "A Parent Guide to Adolescent Depression"

Module 1: Getting Started, Session 2

Outline of Session

ADOLESCENT ONLY

Check-In

- Complete the SMFQ/PHQ-9.
- Review the SMFQ/PHQ-9.
- Generate Today's Agenda, including the allocation of time to review session material, as well as the Adolescent's Agenda items.

"Test It Out" Review: Handout 3 (Test It Out): "Activity Monitoring"

"Let's review your activity monitoring from last week [complete if the adolescent did not finish it]. Did you notice any surprises in what you were doing? Did the day seem typical for you? If not, what was different?"

Key Concepts for Today's Session

"The rationale for today's session is to begin to talk about how our relationships and activities in our life impact our mood, and how our mood, in turn, impacts our actions and ultimately the way we feel."

Concept 1: How Relationships and Activities Impact Mood

"To get a sense of different relationships and activities in your life, let's talk through this worksheet together. In particular, I would like to hear more about the most important people and activities in your life and how they increase or decrease your depression."

Introduce Handout 4 (Worksheet): "Who and What Is on 'First' in Your Life?"

- Using the visual provided (Handout 4), orient the adolescent to the concentric circles. *"At the center of this diagram is you. I would like to ask you to indicate, with a 'dot,' different people and activities that you consider to be important in your life. The closer you mark them toward the center (you), the more important they are. As you do this, please know that 'important' can be considered either positively or negatively. For example, you might say, 'Horseback riding is important,' but you may really dislike it, and it is only important because your mom and dad make you engage in it for 5 hours every week. On the other hand, you might place a dot for your aunt and note that she is important because you enjoy spending time with her and she does fun activities with you, like going to the movies. Last, you should know that you can also put people or activities on here that you are missing—like if you have lost someone or you are no longer doing an activity. It is good to note those things because they, too, impact your mood. So . . . who and what is on 'first' in your life?"*

- Make sure that this is an interactive process and learn about each "dot" as you go along. It is fine for the therapist to serve as the scribe if that makes completing this task smoother and more interactive. Help the adolescent to take the lead as much as possible, and use the following questions as a guide:
    - *"Who would you identify as 'your important people' and what would you identify as 'your important activities'?"*
    - *"If you were to rate their level of importance, how and where would you rate them?"* (Use this to help place people and activities on the circle.)
    - *"What makes one person or activity more important than another?"*
    - *"What people and activities contribute most to your depression and why?"*
    - *"What people and activities reduce your depression, and how so?"*
    - *"Is there anyone or anything in your life that you are missing? How does that increase or reduce your depression?"*

Concept 2: The Situation–Activity–Mood Cycle

"Now that we have a better understanding of who and what is on 'first' in your life, let's build on that and begin to talk about drawing connections among situations that occur, our response and what we do, and the impact on our mood. When we draw these connections, we can often see what we call 'downward spirals' and 'upward spirals.' We can get into a 'downward spiral' when we respond to a difficult situation in a way that makes our mood worse. For example, when you are waiting to hear from a friend, and you shoot off an angry text, only to find out later that your friend had to turn off her phone in math class, you feel bad. On the other hand, we can get into an 'upward spiral' when we make a funny comment, everyone laughs, and we feel more confident to share more jokes in the future."

Introduce Handout 5 (Test It Out): "Downward Spiral, Upward Spiral"

"This worksheet will begin to help you notice connections between situations, your reaction, what you do and the impact on your mood. Let's work through this together and think of examples in your own life over the last few days. Let's start with the 'downward spiral.' Can you think of a time in which something happened that brought your mood down? Let's talk about what happened, how you reacted and what you did, and whether you felt better or worse. Now let's talk about a time when something happened that brought your mood up. Let's talk about what happened, how you reacted and what you did, and whether you felt better or worse."

- If possible, tie in activities or events the adolescent has included in last week's "Test It Out" activity or experiences the adolescent has shared that are relavant to him or her. Use the adolescent's personal examples and experiences to help the "Downward Spiral, Upward Spiral" exercise make sense.

"Test It Out" for the Coming Week: Introduce (Second Copy) Handout 5 (Test It Out): "Downward Spiral, Upward Spiral"

"Your 'Test It Out' work for the week is to identify two things that happen between now and the next session—one that led to a 'downward spiral' and another that led to an 'upward spiral,' using Handout 5."

- Encourage the adolescent to pay attention to what happened, and write down how he or she felt, what he or she did, and how he or she felt after that.
- Ask the adolescent to bring the worksheet back to the next session so that it can be reviewed and together you can begin to talk about how to learn to use activity to change mood.

Thanks and Next Steps

- Thank the adolescent for his or her participation today and ask if there are further questions you can answer at this time.
- Share that you will briefly meet with his or her parent(s), with the goal of sharing some information about adolescent depression.
- Preview that the next module will focus more on how the adolescent can use activities to improve his or her mood.

PARENT(S) ONLY

"Welcome back and thank you for coming in! Today I want to touch base about a few things. I want to provide you with information about depression in adolescence and offer suggestions related to how you might support your son or daughter as he or she begins to get more 'active' in life."

Ask the parent(s) whether they have any questions and then answer any questions that come up.

Key Concepts for Today's Session

Concept 1: Depression in Adolescence

"Let's start today by talking more specifically about depression and what it means for your son or daughter."

Introduce Handout 6 (Teaching Guide): "A Parent Guide to Adolescent Depression"

"Here is a handout entitled 'A Parent Guide to Adolescent Depression.' You can take it with you and review it; however, I would like to discuss a few key points and concepts that are covered in the handout."

- *"For starters, every teen is a bit different, but common symptoms of depression you may have noticed in your son or daughter include things like _____."*
- Highlight symptoms of depression that they may have noticed in their adolescent in the past or currently, including the following:
    - Depressed or irritable mood
    - Anhedonia or lack of interest/pleasure in usual activities
    - Appetite or weight difficulties/changes
    - Sleep difficulties or changes (too much, too little, poor)
    - Fatigue
    - Excessive guilt
    - Concentration difficulties
    - Suicidal ideation or behavior
- Also highlight associated symptoms, including the following:
    - Lack of reactivity
    - Hopelessness/helplessness
    - Anxiety
    - Somatic complaints
    - Oppositionality
- *"Depression in teens is very common."*
    - Discuss the fact that their teen is not alone and the idea that depression is very common. On any given day in the United States, approximately 2–5% of adolescents are struggling with some kind of depressive episode. By the time teens graduate from high school (age 18), about 20% have had a depressive episode at some point in time.
- *"Treatment is very important."*
    - Discuss the importance of treatment, the idea that depression does seem to respond to treatment, and that while treatment takes time, it does seem to have the benefit of shortening the length of the depressive episode.
    - Discuss the idea that doing things to decrease the length of the depressive episode (e.g., engaging in treatment) is important because we know that depression affects academic, social, and family functioning.
- *"While the exact cause of depression is likely somewhat different for different teens, it is clear that stress plays a key role in the onset and maintenance of depression over time."*
    - Highlight that there are many different theories of depression, all of which seem to have some research evidence behind them, and that while there are many pathways (causes) to the same outcome (depressive symptoms), the role of stress (e.g., academic pressures, problems with peers, changes at puberty, family conflict) in the onset and maintenance of depression cannot be underestimated.
    - Highlight the importance of regular sleeping patterns and good sleep hygiene, as well as exercise, in managing depressive symptoms over time.

- *"Parenting a teen is challenging in good times, and it can be extraordinarily heartbreaking in the face of depression. It is not only difficult to see your child go through such difficult times and feel so sad, but it can even be more challenging when your teen is irritable, angry, and oppositional toward you."*
- Validate the parent's experiences and how challenging it can be to parent an adolescent who is struggling with depression. Remind them that these are common symptoms, and encourage the parent(s) to try to separate their teen's behavior from their self-worth as parent(s). To this end, encourage them to reframe their teen's behavior as his or her depression talking, and highlight the importance of responding with warmth and understanding rather than anger and disdain, which will only reinforce ongoing negative interactions.

Recap of Adolescent Session Concepts

Briefly review the concepts discussed in this session with the adolescent:

- In addition to events in our environment, relationships/activities impact our mood.
- It is important to notice the connections between situations and our responses—what we do (activity) and how we feel (mood).
- Our actions can maintain, improve, or worsen our mood.
- We can get into a "downward spiral" when we react to a situation by doing something that brings down our mood and/or worsens the original problem.
- We can get into an "upward spiral" when we react to a situation by doing something that improves our mood and leads to more effective coping.
- Once we can recognize the pattern of the spiral that the adolescent is in, we will begin to teach the adolescent how to use activity to change his or her mood.

Concept 2: Supporting Your Adolescent through His or Her Depression

"We have talked about a lot of important things today. Before we wrap up, I want to highlight a few more things and specifically talk about how to support your teen through his or her depression. As part of the A-BAP, we will ask you to do the following:

- *Encourage your adolescent. Don't nag, but encourage him or her to use the concepts we discuss.*
- *The challenge is to do so without getting frustrated, upset, angry, or mad, as we previously discussed.*
- *While more detail will follow, some initial ideas include:*
  - *Validate your adolescent's feelings.*
  - *Attempt to reduce stress.*
  - *Be realistic in your expectations for your adolescent while he or she is dealing with depression.*
  - *Support him or her in getting active, even if it comes at a bit of a cost (e.g., providing transportation, providing reasonable finances)."*

Thanks and Next Steps

- Thank the parent(s) for their participation today and ask whether there are further questions you can answer at this time.
- Preview that in the next session, you will continue to talk about their experiences and concerns as the parent(s) of an adolescent who is coping with depression.

MODULE 2
Getting Active

SESSION 3

Goal-Directed Behavior versus Mood-Directed Behavior

Suggested Total Session Time: 50–60 minutes

Session Overview

Goals

This module centers on a more in-depth discussion of how "getting active," even when adolescents are feeling down, can help them begin to feel better. There are two main goals for Session 3:

1. Introduce the BA concept regarding the role of activation in mood management, specifically mood-directed behavior versus goal-directed behavior, and the importance of using action to help oneself feel better rather than waiting to feel better before increasing activity.
2. Provide psychoeducational information to the parent(s) about adolescent depression.

Structure and Teaching Points

This module is structured to include a working session with the adolescent, followed by a brief check-in and teaching exercise with the parent(s). Introduce the following core teaching concepts:

- Moods are inextricably connected to what we do—some activities make us feel better, while other activities make us feel worse.
- When we are feeling down, it is important *not* to wait to feel better before doing something (e.g., it is important not to engage in **mood-directed behavior**); getting active when we are feeling down (e.g., engaging in **goal-directed behavior**) may help us begin to get out of the vicious cycle of depression.
- The A-BAP asks people to act first, then to observe, *over time,* whether the action improves mood.
- A first step toward engaging in goal-directed behavior centers on gaining a better understanding of what activities help us feel better, and the best way to do this involves monitoring and paying attention to the links among the situations in our environment, our activities, and our moods.
- Tracking what is happening around you (situations), what you do (activities), and how it affects your mood will help you learn to differentiate activities that help you feel better versus activities that get you down.
- With the parent(s), continue to provide some psychoeducation about depression through discussion of last week's homework, as well as engage parent(s) in a brief exercise designed to validate their experiences, both positive and challenging, of parenting an adolescent who is struggling with depression.

Session Agenda

Adolescent Only

- Check-In
- Key Concepts for today's session:
  - Concept 1: Using Activity to Improve Mood
    - Handout 7 (Teaching Guide): "Getting Active!"
  - Concept 2: Activity–Mood Monitoring
    - Handout 8 (Worksheet): "Activity–Mood Chart—Example"
- "Test It Out" activity for the week: Handout 9 (Test It Out): "Activity–Mood Chart"

Parent(s) Only

- Key Concepts for today's session:
  - Concept 1: Supporting Your Adolescent Who Is Struggling with Depression
    - Handout 10 (Worksheet): "Ways to Describe Parenting an Adolescent"

Materials You Need to Have Ready

- Today's Agenda
- SMFQ/PHQ-9
- Handout 5 (Test It Out): "Downward Spiral, Upward Spiral"
- Handout 6 (Test It Out): "A Parent Guide to Adolescent Depression"
- Handout 7 (Teaching Guide): "Getting Active!"
- Handout 8 (Worksheet): "Activity–Mood Chart—Example"
- Handout 9 (Test It Out): "Activity–Mood Chart"
- Handout 10 (Worksheet): "Ways to Describe Parenting an Adolescent"

Outline of Session

ADOLESCENT ONLY

Check-In

- Complete the SMFQ/PHQ-9.
- Review the SMFQ/PHQ-9.
- Generate Today's Agenda, including the allocation of time to review session material, as well as the Adolescent's Agenda items.

"Test It Out" Review: Handout 5: "Downward Spiral, Upward Spiral"

"Let's review your 'Downward Spiral, Upward Spiral' [complete it if the adolescent did not finish it]. Can you see how what you did in a situation affected how you felt, either good or bad? Do you think that led to other behaviors or actions? As you look at it now, is there something you would have done differently?"

Key Concepts for Today's Session

"The rationale for today's session is to talk more about how moods are connected to what we do. By this, I mean that we cannot separate moods from the activities we engage in—some activities make us feel better, and other activities make us feel worse. The secret in all of this is that we can use activities and behaviors to control or regulate our mood."

Concept 1: Using Activity to Improve Mood

"Let's start today by talking about how we can use activity to improve our mood. Do you remember the last session when we talked about 'upward and downward spirals'? We were already starting to draw connections to the idea that some activities, behaviors, or things that we do make us feel better and other activities, behaviors, or things that we do make us feel worse."

Introduce Handout 7 (Teaching Guide): "Getting Active!"

"Let's look at this handout ('Getting Active!'). Here you can see three examples. The first two examples are of something called mood-directed behavior, and the third example is of something called goal-directed behavior."

- Review the three examples with the adolescent.
  - *"In the first example, the person is feeling down, does nothing, and he or she feels worse. This is an example of mood-directed behavior.*
  - *In the second example, the person is feeling happy, does something fun and feels even better. This is also an example of mood-directed behavior.*
  - *In the third example, the person is feeling down but does something fun anyway and ends up feeling a bit better. This is an example of goal-directed behavior."*
- Highlight key teaching points in the handout:
  - *"The idea here is that instead of waiting to feel better before doing something which is mood-directed behavior you do something, knowing that it may eventually help you get out of your cycle of depression which is goal-directed behavior.*
  - *If you wait to be less depressed and more motivated before engaging in activities that make you feel less depressed and more motivated, you may wait for a long time and will stay stuck.*
  - *Waiting to feel more motivated before changing your behavior is not likely to be an effective strategy.*
  - *The A-BAP asks you to act first, and observe over time, whether the action improves mood. The idea is that your goal (feeling better) should dictate your activities rather than your mood (feeling crappy, so you do nothing)."*

In-Session Exercise

Practice the concept of goal-directed behavior with the adolescent by modeling or doing it with him or her.

- Rate mood on a scale of 1–10 ("10" is high).
- Engage in brief (30–60 seconds) activity (e.g., watch a YouTube video, listen to a favorite upbeat song, listen to a brief comedy routine, take a brisk walk around your setting, engage in a breathing exercise or yoga pose).
- Rate mood again on a scale of 1–10 ("10" is high).
- Discuss what happened. If there is no change or if it makes the adolescent feel worse, remind him or her that change takes time, and that you will ultimately be discussing activities that are effective for him or her; acknowledge that it was useful information, no matter what. If there is a change, highlight that this is part of what goal-directed behavior is all about and share that you will both keep experimenting and find other activities that can be useful.

Concept 2: Activity–Mood Monitoring

"While changing your activity can help to change your mood, the fact remains that it is sometimes difficult to know where to start. The first step is to begin to pay attention to the links between the activities and moods in your daily life. One of the best ways to pay attention to what activities are effective in helping to shift our moods centers on keeping track of what we are doing and how we are feeling."

Introduce Handout 8 (Worksheet): "Activity–Mood Chart—Example"

- Walk through the example on the left of the chart with the adolescent: *"Now that you have seen the example, let's see if you can complete this for the hours prior to your appointment today. We can walk through it together."*
- Try to elicit as much detail as possible about what the teen was doing, and the corresponding moods/feelings.
- Questions that help reinforce the teen noticing relations between activity and mood include the following:
  - *"When you were doing X, how did you feel?"*
  - *"Did you notice a change, **even a very small one**?"*
  - *"Did you notice a change, **even for just a few minutes**?"*
  - *"What were you doing when you felt that way?"*
  - *"Where were you at the time that such a feeling occurred?"*
  - *"If you had been doing Y instead of Z, how would you have felt?"*
- Once you have two situations in which the adolescent reports a significant mood change, you can begin to discuss the patterns and point out the links.
- Point out that there is a connection between what the adolescent does and associated feelings in as many places as you can by observing mood shifts noted in Handout 8: "Activity–Mood Chart—Example".
- Help the adolescent identify links between activity and mood (e.g., feeling sad lying in bed after school, feeling energized when riding bike after school). Highlight the following:
  - *"You can learn what sorts of activities may be effective and could be done more frequently."*
  - *"You can learn what sorts of activities are bringing you down, which can be addressed in future sessions as coping strategies are discussed."*

"Test It Out" for the Coming Week: Introduce Handout 9 (Test It Out): "Activity–Mood Chart"

"Your 'Test It Out' work for the week is to monitor your activities and the associated moods using the Activity–Mood Chart (Handout 9). This chart is just like the sample chart (Handout 8: 'Activity–Mood Chart—Example') we just completed. I want you to

pick 2 days to focus on—choose a school day and a weekend day—so we can see if there is any difference." Review what you want the adolescent to practice over the week to make sure that he or she understands.

Thanks and Next Steps

"I am going to meet briefly with your parent(s) to touch base, provide some information about depression [or whatever term the teen uses to refer to his or her mood difficulties], *and review the idea that you can use activity to control or regulate mood as we've discussed today."*

- Assure the adolescent that issues that have come up in your meeting will not be discussed unless he or she requests that they do.
- Preview that the next module will get more specific regarding activities that will be effective to help the adolescent manage mood both in the short term and the long run.

PARENT(S) ONLY

Concept 1: Supporting Your Adolescent Who Is Struggling with Depression

"Welcome back! Today I want to touch base about a few things. First and foremost I want to see if you have any questions about 'A Parent Guide to Adolescent Depression,' which I gave you during our last session. Then I want to talk with you a bit about how to best support an adolescent struggling with depression. Let's start with the handout. Do you have any questions or concerns about what you read?"

- Ask the parent(s) if they have any questions regarding Handout 6: "A Parent Guide to Adolescent Depression" and answer any questions they might have.

Introduce Handout 10 (Worksheet): "Ways to Describe Parenting an Adolescent"

- Using Handout 10 (Worksheet): "Ways to Describe Parenting an Adolescent," ask the parent(s) to circle the words that best describe their experience parenting an adolescent. Ask them to talk a bit about some of the words they have selected.
- Spend a few moments talking about what has been hard in parenting their adolescent with depression, using the words that they have circled.
- Highlight that they are not alone—that other parents of adolescents struggling with depression have told you similar things and also find their parenting experience to be one that is important, challenging, and fun, but also frustrating (use their words as you discuss this).
- Validate their experience and acknowledge that because adolescents with depression

can be so irritable, angry, and oppositional, it is often difficult to stay focused on how best to support them.
- Explain that their adolescent's behavior is a function of being depressed.

For example, if working with the parent of an adolescent like our case example, Rebecca, you might say: *"You circled the whole worksheet—parenting Rebecca is very complicated! It must have been so hard to go from having a fun and loving little girl to a more challenging and confusing teenager. With the emergence of her depression, it sounds as though you felt you lost her, but with treatment of her depression, including getting the right kind of support from you, we expect that you will once again see those parts of your daughter that you've missed and you can help her to learn how to structure her life to stave off future bouts of depression."*

Thanks and Next Steps

Thank the parent(s) for their participation today and ask if there are further questions you can answer at this time. Preview that the next parent session will continue with a discussion of specifics about supporting their adolescent with depression.

SESSION 4

Introducing Consequences of Behavior

Suggested Total Session Time: 50–60 minutes

Session Overview

Goals

Session 4 centers on functional analysis and helping adolescents understand why they do what they do. There are three main goals in this session:

1. Help the adolescent realize that some activities will make him or her feel better, that others will make him or her feel worse, and that inactivity will maintain depressive symptoms.
2. Assist the adolescent in understanding his or her behavior patterns and help the adolescent appreciate that his or her behaviors make sense in particular situations given the outcomes typically experienced.
3. Teach the adolescent to question his or her behavior and to consider it in terms of immediate and longer-term consequences.

Structure and Teaching Points

This session is structured to include a working session with the adolescent only. The main points are as follows:

Module 2: Getting Active, Session 4

- Introduce functional analysis, addressing the following points:
  - Behavior that is reinforced (e.g., makes us feel good, brings us relief) usually gets repeated, but it may not always help us reach our longer-term goals and objectives.
  - There is a payoff and price to all behaviors/activities. We do things when there is a payoff, and we do not do other things when there is a price.
- Consider the short- and long-term consequences of the behavior/activity.
- Identify activities that affect mood: "Pump You Up" and "Bring You Down" activities.
- Make the most of good feelings.

Session Agenda

Adolescent Only

- Check-In
- Key Concepts for today's session:
  - Concept 1: Functional Analysis: Payoff versus Price—Why We Do What We Do
  - Concept 2: Short-Term versus Long-Term Consequences
  - Handout 11 (Teaching Guide): "Short- versus Long-Term Consequences"
  - Concept 3. "Pump You Up" versus "Bring You Down" activities
    - Handout 12 (Worksheet): "Pump You Up, Bring You Down" and Handout 13 (Teaching Guide): "Activities Menu"
  - Concept 4: Making the Most of a Good Feeling
- "Test It Out" activity for the week: Handout 14 (Test It Out): "Activities That Help to PUMP You UP!!"

Materials You Need to Have Ready

- Today's Agenda
- SMFQ/PHQ-9
- Handout 9 (Test It Out): "Activity–Mood Chart"
- Handout 11 (Teaching Guide): "Short- versus Long-Term Consequences"
- Handout 12 (Worksheet): "Pump You Up, Bring You Down"
- Handout 13 (Teaching Guide): "Activities Menu"
- Handout 14 (Test It Out): "Activities That Help to PUMP You UP!!"

Outline of Session

ADOLESCENT ONLY

Check-In

- Complete the SMFQ/PHQ-9.
- Review the SMFQ/PHQ-9.
- Generate Today's Agenda, including the allocation of time to review session material, as well as the Adolescent's Agenda items.

"Test It Out" Review: Handout 9: "Activity–Mood Chart"

Review/complete Handout 9 ("Activity–Mood Chart") and emphasize any patterns or connection between activities and any associated mood changes for the adolescent.

Key Concepts for Today's Session

"The rationale for today's session is to talk more about 'why we do what we do' and figure out what works best in the long run to help us feel better and be more effective. You've told me you really like to _____ [insert adolescent's interest; e.g., listening to music]. What do you like about that activity? Most people do the things they do because of what happens after they do them. That is, they do what they do because of the 'consequences' of their actions. When we hear the word consequences, *we often think negatively, but consequences can also be positive. For example, we often do what we do because doing it makes us feel better."*

Concept 1: Functional Analysis: Payoff versus Price—Why We Do What We Do

"Let's start today by talking about something called 'functional analysis,' which is a fancy term for understanding behavior and why we do what we do. In general, we tend to do certain things because there is a 'payoff,' and we tend not to do other things because they come with a 'price.'"

- The payoff: *"More specifically, we usually do things because the payoff is good. For instance, we might spend time on the computer in the evening because it is fun and it allows us to get in touch with other people or play a game we like. Can you think of some things that you do because the payoff is good?"*
- The price: *"If the price of our action is too high, however, we probably won't do it again. So, with the computer example, we know that it can turn from feeling like a payoff to feeling like we are paying a price if we stay up too late on the computer, get to bed much later than usual, and end up feeling really tired and grumpy in the morning.*

We might think twice before doing that again. Can you think of some things that you do not do because of the price?"

- Using material the adolescent has brought up in session, find an example that you can use to discuss the payoff and price of different behaviors/activities.

Concept 2: Short-Term versus Long-Term Consequences

"When thinking about the 'payoff' and 'price' of certain behavior it is also important to consider how we balance short- and long-term consequences of our behavior. More specifically, some behaviors have both a short- and a long-term payoff, while others have both a short- and long-term price; still others are mixed."

Introduce Handout 11 (Teaching Guide):
"Short- versus Long-Term Consequences"

"Many activities come with their own rewards right away—if you see a great movie with friends one evening, then you are likely to have a positive mood that night. But sometimes activities that will help your mood over time don't immediately feel great. For example, practicing chords on your guitar can be very boring and also hurt your fingers. In this case, the immediate result of this activity involves a price, but, over time, it pays off since you can learn to play your favorite songs or jam with friends.

The opposite situation is also tricky. Problems arise with activities that have an immediate or short-term payoff but a long-term price. Here are some examples:

- *Borrowing money to buy an expensive game brings the immediate satisfaction of having the game, but the long-term price of owing money and having to pay it back.*
- *Smoking pot may make you feel good in the moment, but in the long term it decreases motivation, negatively affects grades, and may lead to trouble with the law."*

"So let's walk through some of the activities you like to think about how they line up in terms of both short- and long-term payoffs."

Use Handout 11 (Teaching Guide): "Short- versus Long-Term Consequences" to evaluate the payoff and price of some activities the adolescent likes or avoids. Walk through possible pros and cons of behavioral choices.

Make sure to integrate the concepts (choosing activities, functional analysis, and short- vs. long-term consequences). *"For example, a chosen activity may improve your mood in the short term (payoff) but brings you down in the long term (price). Another activity, like studying for a test, might bring you down in the short term but the long-term payoff, getting a good grade, may be worth it. Ultimately, it's important to consider both the short- and long-term payoff and price."*

Concept 3: "Pump You Up" versus "Bring You Down" Activities

"Now that we have an understanding of functional assessment and the short- and long-term payoff and price of certain behaviors, let's talk about another concept. While we cannot always control the situations we find ourselves in, we can try to choose activities that will help us feel better. Activities generally fall into two categories: 'Pump You Up' and 'Bring You Down.' Let's look at some of the things that you do on a typical day and see if we can figure out their category."

- Help the teen list specific activities, not just contexts and events (e.g., a "Bring You Down" activity listed as "being at home" would be more effectively stated as "arguing with my mother about chores").
- Discuss examples of "Pump You Up" and "Bring You Down" activities that have already been discussed over the course of therapy. For example, with an adolescent whose only interest is video games, initial discussions about "Pump You Up" activities may focus on the limited topic of video games, with attention to ideas about how to improve the enjoyment of these games and ideas for new games. This could provide a platform for commenting on how these behaviors/activities might improve mood even if he or she cannot identify any "Pump You Up" activities on his or her own.

Introduce Handout 12 (Worksheet): "Pump You Up, Bring You Down"

"Let's look at some of the things that you do on a typical day and see in which category they fall." Use Handout 12 to generate a list of "Pump You Up" and "Bring You Down" activities. (*Note.* It may also be helpful to review the adolescent's "Test It Out" material from Sessions 2 and 3.)

Introduce Handout 13 (Teaching Guide): "Activities Menu"

"I want to show you a list of 'Pump You Up' activities. Some of these activities might already be on your list, while there may be others that you have never thought of before. I like to introduce adolescents to them because I think they show a number of really interesting things to keep in mind. For example, I think that in looking through them you will see the following:

- *Activities come in all shapes and sizes.*
- *Some activities are short (moments) and others are long (hours).*
- *There are a lot of activities you can do on your own without another person or any special equipment.*
- *Many activities are free, but some require money.*
- *Some activities simply allow you to 'savor' what you value."*

Concept 4: Making the Most of a Good Feeling

"It is important to make the most of good feelings and take the time to really experience and enjoy times when you are feeling good. This is especially important when feeling down or stressed out because thinking about good times can help improve your mood when you are feeling down."

- Encourage the adolescent to do a brief experiment with you in session:
    - Ask him or her to do a quick rating of his or her current mood.
    - Then ask him or her to think of a time when he or she was happily engaged in a favorite activity—have him or her describe who they were with, as well as the sounds, smells, colors, and place of the activity, and last, what made it enjoyable.
    - Walk through with the adolescent what he or she was doing and what about that activity contributed to the good feeling—physical activity, being with friends, reading a good book, and so forth.
    - Help him or her to articulate what it was that contributed to feeling good.
    - Help the adolescent bask in the "good" feeling for just a few minutes, then do another mood rating.
- Teach the adolescent how to use "attention to experience" when enjoying him- or herself, which means paying attention to who they are with, the sounds, the smells, the colors, the place, the feelings, and other details.
- Also talk about ways to extend the experience—take photos, text a friend, make a journal entry, draw a cartoon or picture, post it on Facebook, and so forth.
- Introduce the idea of thinking back to good times as a way to improve mood when feeling low. Encourage the adolescent to try to see whether remembering/thinking about a good time improves his or her mood.
- Stress the need to ***structure carefully*** and avoid setting up disappointment (e.g., if an adolescent suggests that he or she felt happy when his or her boyfriend/girlfriend was around and they have since broken up).

"Test It Out" for the Coming Week: Introduce Handout 14 (Test It Out): "Activities that Help to PUMP You UP!!"

"Before we end today, let's think about the coming week and schedule one or two activities that you know have 'pumped you up' in the past and have improved your mood. Let's try to focus on activities that not only have the short-term payoff of 'pumping you up' but also a long-term payoff. We definitely do not want to select anything that has a long-term price! For example, smoking pot might 'pump you up,' but it would not be an activity to schedule, since the long-term price is likely to outweigh the short-term payoff."

"Your 'Test It Out' work for the week is to keep track of these activities and monitor their effect on your mood. Also, practice 'making the most of good feelings' by identifying a time you felt good, even for a few minutes. Let's identify three things you might try to hold on to that good feeling, like texting a friend or taking a picture. Keep track of it on your 'Test It Out' form over the course of the week."

Thanks and Next Steps

"Before we end today, I want to make sure you do not have any questions."

Preview that the next module will focus on problem solving and figuring out how to handle challenging situations and managing stress.

MODULE 3
Skill Building

SESSION 5

Problem Solving

Suggested Total Session Time: 50–60 minutes

Session Overview

Goals

Session 5 centers on problem solving. Goals of this session are as follows:

1. Review the role of stress as a trigger for depression.
2. Discuss contexts in which it can be useful to use a problem-solving framework, such as stressful or difficult situations.
3. Teach the adolescent a problem-solving framework (COPE), including calming and relaxation strategies.
4. Teach the parent(s) about how to communicate with support, including active listening skills; provide the parent(s) an opportunity to practice supportive communication.

Structure and Teaching Points

This module is structured to include a working session with the adolescent, followed by a more extensive teaching exercise with the parent(s). In this session it is recommended that at least half of the time be allotted to the parent(s). The main teaching points are as follows:

- Introduce the core teaching concept(s):
  - Using problem-solving skills is important when you are stressed, upset, or are having trouble making a decision.
  - There are four basic steps to problem solving (COPE): (1) Calm and Clarify, (2) Options, (3) Pick and Perform, and (4) Evaluate.
- Close the session by introducing the Session 5 "Test It Out."
- Transition to working with the parent(s), allowing time to address their questions and concerns, and engage parent(s) with information related to tools for communication support related to the goal of "getting active."

Session Agenda

Adolescent Only

- Check-In
- Key Concept for today's session:
  - Concept 1: Using COPE to Handle Challenging Situations and Manage Stress
    - Handout 15 (Teaching Guide): "Using COPE to Solve Problems"
- "Test It Out" activity for the week: Handout 16 (Test It Out): "Using COPE"

Parent(s) Only

- Key Concept for today's session:
  - Concept 1: Communication Tools—Active Listening
    - Handout 17 (Teaching Guide): "How to Communicate with Support"
    - Handout 18 (Worksheet): "Practicing How to Communicate with Support"
    - Handout 19 (Test It Out): "Communicating with Support: What Can You Do to Help an Interaction Go Well?"

Materials You Need to Have Ready

- Today's Agenda
- SMFQ/PHQ-9
- Handout 14 (Test It Out): "Activities That Help to PUMP You UP!!"
- Handout 15 (Teaching Guide): "Using COPE to Solve Problems"
- Handout 16 (Test It Out): "Using COPE"
- Handout 17 (Teaching Guide): "How to Communicate with Support"
- Handout 18 (Worksheet): "Practicing How to Communicate with Support"
- Handout 19 (Test It Out): "Communicating with Support: What Can You Do to Help an Interaction Go Well?"

Module 3: Skill Building, Session 5

Outline of Session

ADOLESCENT ONLY

Check-In

- Complete the SMFQ/PHQ-9.
- Review the SMFQ/PHQ-9.
- Generate Today's Agenda, including the allocation of time to review session material, as well as the Adolescent's Agenda items.

"Test It Out" Review: Handout 14: "Activities That Help to PUMP You UP!!"

- Review/complete Handout 14 and focus on whether the adolescent completed a "pump you up activity." In this review, discuss the following:
  - How it impacted his or her mood.
  - The payoff or price.
  - The short-term or long-term consequences.
  - The adolescent's experience in "making the most of a good feeling."
- Discuss how to ensure that the adolescent continues to engage in activities that were effective, as well as how to continue to expand his or her repertoire and/or the frequency of such activities.

Key Concept for Today's Session

*"It is great that you tried some 'pump you up' activities. Sometimes, however, figuring out what to do is easier said than done, especially in a challenging or stressful situation. Today we are going to talk about how you figure out what you want to do when faced with a challenging or stressful situation. Feeling 'stressed out' is a **common** trigger for spiraling down into depression. But life is full of things that can make us feel stressed—exams, arguments with parents or friends, money worries. None of us can avoid stress, but we can learn ways to handle it."*

Concept 1: Using COPE to Handle Challenging Situations and Manage Stress

"Stress can come in many forms—there are big events, like _____ [insert the adolescent's example, e.g., parents' divorce, loss of a pet, moving], but stress also shows up with little hassles like _____ [insert the adolescent's example; e.g., an annoying sibling, pop quizzes, getting a cold]. When we feel stressed, it is easy to act too quickly or impulsively, and we end up doing something that we later regret and has a long-term price for us. For example, talking back to your teacher in a moment of frustration may come with a long-term price. Because of this, it's important to have a strategy to manage

stressful situations. One important step in handling stress is to stop to figure out what the problem really is before reacting."

Introduce Handout 15 (Teaching Guide):
"Using COPE to Solve Problems"

"You already solve many problems every day, without even thinking about it—like whether to wear shorts or jeans to school. But figuring out what to do when you feel stressed or angry can be more difficult. We have found that it is helpful to have a strategy or a plan when faced with something really hard or stressful. Our plan is called COPE, and there are four basic steps within this problem-solving framework."

- Point out that most of us have *triggers*—situations, feelings, or people that give rise to strong emotions. *"It is easy to respond to these triggers in a way that can get you in trouble or make the problem worse. Like sending an angry text to a friend without knowing the full story, or talking back to a teacher who treats you unfairly. Most of us have specific triggers that can spike a sad or angry feeling; what we do next is critical."* Ask the adolescent to name a few of his or her key triggers or help him or her identify these based on the things you have been talking about in therapy.
- *"Let's walk through the COPE approach."* Ask the adolescent to share a problem he or she had in the last week. If the adolescent is unable to do so, provide an example such as the following: The adolescent is feeling uptight because he or she is expecting a call from a friend. He or she thought the friend would call over 2 hours ago and is feeling sad and rejected, and may believe that this friend may not like him or her after all. The adolescent's mother reminds him that it is 9:00 P.M. and time to put the cell phone away for the evening. The adolescent's impulse is to yell at his or her mother.

STEP 1: CALM AND CLARIFY

- **Getting calm**—*"Let's talk about some ways to get yourself calm again when your feelings take over."* Remind the adolescent to pay attention to how he or she is feeling (e.g., angry, scared) and what his or her body is telling him or her (e.g., feeling hot, stomach churning).
  - **Counting**—*"To give yourself a minute to calm down if you are angry and about to do or say something you may regret, STOP and COUNT SLOWLY to 5 or 10."*
  - **Breathing**—*"Another thing you can do is focus on your breathing pattern. Focusing on breathing deeply and slowly can counteract your body's tendency to tense up and help you feel more relaxed, so you can think clearly. To do this, start by taking a breath in, inhaling through your nose, and counting to three slowly then exhaling— EVEN MORE SLOWLY . . . counting to 5."*
  - **Muscle relaxation**—*"Another thing you can do is practice tensing up then relaxing your muscles. This, too, tells your body to calm down rather than stay on alert. You*

can do this in a really easy way by clenching and then opening your hands . . . or you can find a quiet place and practice relaxing all your muscles."
- **Distraction strategies**—"*You can listen to calming music or imagine a place that is really relaxing and happy for you.*"

You can walk the adolescent through this in as much detail as needed.

- Clarifying what the problem really is—"*Taking a minute to CALM down is the crucial first step. When you are calm and thinking clearly you can take a minute to **clarify** what the problem really is, name it, then maintain your calm while sorting out what action you want to take.*"
  - Again, provide examples or build on examples given earlier to demonstrate that your first assessment of what is upsetting you may not always be right. "*For instance, when you have the impulse to yell at your mother, you might be thinking she is the problem, but if you think a minute, you might discover that you are really sad and feeling rejected because your friend did not call you back.*"

STEP 2: GENERATE OPTIONS

- Generate as many options as possible. "*Now that you've clarified the problem, let's take a few minutes to identify all possible options available—let's just throw them all out on the table even if they seem silly or like long shots.*"
- Examine the payoff and price/short-term versus long-term consequences of the options. "*STEPS 3 and 4 involve taking an action, then observing whether it worked for you.*

STEP 3: PERFORM

- Pick a solution. "*Based on our list of options and their price–payoff, what do you think would have been the best one to try?*"
- Anticipate obstacles. "*What could get in the way of trying your option? What can you do to overcome this obstacle?*"
- Try it out. "*Okay, that sounds good.*"

STEP 4: EVALUATE

- Teach the adolescent how to evaluate whether the option worked. Have him or her focus on how the option impacted his or her mood, whether the option had a "payoff" or a "price," and whether it was associated with any "short-term or long-term consequences."
- Highlight that if the option worked, he or she should keep it up.
- Suggest that if the option did not work, the adolescent should revisit his or her OPTIONS list and come up with a different solution.

"Test It Out" for the Coming Week: Introduce Handout 16 (Test It Out):
"Using COPE"

"Your 'Test It Out' work for the week is to use COPE and keep track of how it went using Handout 16, the "Using COPE" form. Complete all parts of the form and record the situation, your responses (including what you felt emotionally and in your body), and what you did using the COPE steps. Keep the COPE sheet handy—pull it out if you run into one of your triggers and use it to help you figure out what you want to do OR if no trigger situations come up, simply practice using COPE with a smaller problem.

"I will ask you what happened at our next session—it will be helpful to know exactly what happened even if it went poorly, because that will allow us to do more problem solving and identify another, likely better option."

Thanks and Next Steps

- Let the adolescent know that you will briefly meet with his or her parent(s) to provide some information about ways to become a good listener.
- Assure the adolescent that issues that have come up in your meeting will not be discussed, unless the adolescent requests that they do.
- Preview that the next session will focus on figuring out how to set good goals.

PARENT(S) ONLY

"Welcome back! Today I wanted to touch base about a few things. Last time we met, we had a chance to talk about what it's like to parent a teen with depression. Today I want to talk about some strategies to communicate and support your teen."

Ask the parent(s) whether they have any questions, and, if so, answer any questions they might have.

Key Concept for Today's Session

Concept 1: Communication Tools—Active Listening

Provide the parent(s) with information regarding tools for communication support in relation to the goal of "getting active."

"Support can come in a lot of forms and, as we discussed last time we met, it can be difficult to provide the type of support that a depressed teen is responsive to, particularly when you are not sure what he or she wants or needs. Sometimes our gut instinct about what support looks like clashes with what the teen is wanting. And each individual needs to be supported differently! This has led us to think about support as something that needs to be discussed and clarified. The first step in determining how to support your teen is to be an active listener. What comes to mind when you think about 'active listening'?"

Introduce Handout 17 (Teaching Guide):
"How to Communicate with Support"

- Using Handout 17, review critical elements of Active Listening with the parent(s).
- Highlight the importance of giving the speaker "the floor," and using the following communication techniques:
  - Clarifying questions
  - Reflecting feelings
  - Paraphrasing

"Many parents readily understand the concept of active listening; however, putting it into action can be tricky. We want to take some time now to practice, so that when you have the chance to try this with your teen, you have some ideas about what works for you."

Introduce Handout 18 (Worksheet): "Practicing How to Communicate with Support"

- In thinking about active listening, use Handout 18 to go through the example situations and help the parent(s) generate a response that reflects active listening.
- Engage the parent(s) in discussion of what might make one response not so effective as a show of support and what makes another response more supportive. For example: *"I could imagine being pretty frustrated and concerned if _____ [insert teen's name] came home with a speeding ticket. Prior to saying anything, it is important to take a moment (or possibly longer, if needed) to calm down. It is also helpful to give your adolescent the floor to let him or her say what he or she needs to say before launching into your own reaction. When your teen is talking, it is very important to listen and paraphrase, even though it will be tempting to respond right away. Should we try it? I'll be your son or daughter . . ."*
- Point out that while it sounds easy to use these approaches, we have found that practice is important.
- Emphasize that how you are feeling (angry, worried) will shape your response—so you need to be aware of your own feelings and what you really want to convey to your son or daughter.

Introduce Handout 19 (Test It Out): "Communicating with Support: What Can You Do to Help an Interaction Go Well?"

Ask the parent(s) to complete Handout 19 over the course of the next week, tracking one situation that required support and did not go so well and another that required support and went smoothly. The handout will be reviewed and discussed in the next meeting.

Thanks and Next Steps

- Thank the parent(s) for their participation today and ask if there are further questions you can answer at this time.
- Preview that the next session will focus on a discussion about ways to support their adolescent.

SESSION 6

Goal Setting

Suggested Total Session Time: 50–60 minutes

Session Overview

Goals

Session 6 centers on goal setting. Goals of this module are as follows:

- Introduce adolescents to SMART goals.
- Practice identifying and setting SMART goals.
- Educate the parent(s) on how to support their adolescent better and how to monitor that support.

Structure and Teaching Points

This module is structured to include a working session with the adolescent, followed by a brief check-in and teaching exercise with the parent(s). The main teaching points are as follows:

- The most effective goals are SMART goals—Specific, Measurable, Appealing, Realistic, and Time-Bound.
  - The therapist should ensure that the potential goals being discussed are in an area (e.g., school, sports, social relationships) that the adolescent either values or finds important.
  - Such goal setting will be used to schedule activities in the adolescent's activity

chart and to set the stage for developing tools in future sessions to modify avoidance.
- Difficult goals can be broken into smaller and easier steps (graded task assignment).
  - The adolescent and therapist break down large goals, then agree to have the adolescent try one or two smaller tasks (mini-steps) during the week.
  - Graded task assignments help to address the problem of lack of motivation/interest by helping the adolescent "get active" in small steps.
- Engage parent(s) in education regarding how to support their adolescent and how to monitor that support.

Session Agenda

Adolescent Only

- Check-In
- Key Concept for today's session:
  - Concept 1: Goal Setting
    - Handout 20 (Teaching Guide): "Setting SMART Goals"
    - Handout 21 (Teaching Guide): "How SMART Is This Goal?"
    - Handout 22 (Worksheet): "Identifying a SMART Goal"
- "Test It Out" activity for the week: Handout 23 (Test It Out): "Goal Setting"

Parent(s) Only

- Key Concept for today's session:
  - Concept 1: Providing and Monitoring Support
    - Handout 24 (Teaching Guide): "Ways to Support My Adolescent"
    - Handout 25 (Test It Out): "Monitoring Support"

Materials You Need to Have Ready

- Today's Agenda
- SMFQ/PHQ-9
- Handout 16 (Test It Out): "Using COPE"
- Handout 19 (Test It Out): "Communicating with Support: What You Can Do to Help an Interaction Go Well"
- Handout 20 (Teaching Guide): "Setting SMART Goals"
- Handout 21 (Teaching Guide): "How SMART Is This Goal?"
- Handout 22 (Worksheet): "Identifying a SMART Goal"

- Handout 23 (Test It Out): "Goal Setting"
- Handout 24 (Teaching Guide): "Ways to Support My Adolescent"
- Handout 25 (Test It Out): "Monitoring Support"

Outline of Session

ADOLESCENT ONLY

Check-In

- Complete the SMFQ/PHQ-9.
- Review the SMFQ/PHQ-9.
- Generate Today's Agenda, including the allocation of time to review session material, as well as the Adolescent's Agenda items.

"Test It Out" Review: Handout 16: "Using COPE"

Review/complete Handout 16 ("Using COPE"). Remind the adolescent that the last step in COPE is to *evaluate,* which is what you two are doing together now. Walk through each step and find out what the adolescent did, how it went, and any challenges he or she faced. Emphasize how well it worked for the adolescent, and track what did not go well. Was the adolescent able to identify his or her triggers, feelings, and physical responses; to calm down and generate possible solutions? Use COPE skills if things did not go well and select another OPTION for the adolescent to try. Here are some possible questions/comments to use:

- *"How did it go? What triggers came up that gave you a chance to practice COPE skills?*
- *How did you calm yourself down?*
- *What did you determine the problem to be?*
- *Great list of options—what were the short- and long-term payoffs and prices of each one?"*

Key Concept for Today's Session

"A few sessions ago, we talked about goal-directed versus mood-directed behavior. In that session, we focused on the importance of taking action by engaging in goal-directed behavior as a strategy to improve mood. This is, however, easier said than done. Today, we are going to talk more specifically about how to identify and set goals. Part of doing this includes strategies for choosing goals that are important to you, then being able to break them down into mini-steps so you can accomplish them and not get overwhelmed in the process."

Concept 1: Goal Setting

"One of the first steps in taking action is to take the time to think about what your own goals are—what you would like to work on, accomplish, or change in your life. Today we are going to work on setting a goal—for now, just a short-term goal that is something you can do over this next week that could contribute to helping you feel better."

Introduce Handout 20 (Teaching Guide): "Setting SMART Goals"

- Using Handout 20, begin with the topic of setting SMART goals.
  - Specific—Clear and specifically stated, describing what you will do.
  - Measureable—Identify an easy way to track if the goal was accomplished.
  - Appealing—Desirable, something you value, a healthy choice.
  - Realistic—Achievable, controllable, within reach but not *too* easy.
  - Time-bound—Has a clear start and finish.
- Next, discuss identifying SMART Goals: *"As a first step, let's walk through some examples of goals other adolescents have identified and you can evaluate whether you think they are SMART and meet the criteria we just talked about—that is, if you think the person has a good chance of being successful in reaching this goal."*

Introduce Handout 21 (Teaching Guide): "How SMART Is This Goal?"

- Using Handout 21, go through a few of the "How SMART Is This Goal?" examples and have the adolescent evaluate the goal and talk about how he or she might modify it to improve the chances of a successful outcome. Have the adolescent focus on the SMART acronym.
- Refer back to Handout 20 ("Setting SMART Goals"). *"With each goal, MINI-STEPS are important—if you take on too much at a time, it often interferes with reaching and achieving goals. Once you set your goals, we can work on identifying 'doable' steps you can take each week to ultimately reach your larger goal, and then you can figure out when you could take each step. If barriers to following through should come up, we can talk about ways to overcome them."*
- For example, if the goal is "Do my algebra homework," the first steps may be as simple as (1) get the assignment, (2) bring the book home, (3) review how to do work assigned, and so forth.
- *"Before we start, let's take a minute to think about what is important to you and what may help you feel better or improve your situation."*

Introduce Handout 22 (Worksheet): "Identifying a SMART Goal"

Using Handout 22 ("Identifying a SMART Goal"), ask the adolescent to consider each area of his or her life—school, social, family, activities (sports, band, acting, etc.)—in order to identify the areas in which change would contribute most to feeling better or improving his or her situation.

"Test It Out" for the Coming Week: Introduce Handout 23 (Test It Out): "Goal Setting"

- Once the adolescent has identified the area on which to focus, use Handout 23 (Test It Out): "Goal Setting," and walk him or her through setting a goal, with attention to having the goal be a SMART one. Focus on mini-steps and breaking the goal into "doable" parts, as well as asking the adolescent to schedule a time to complete each mini-step. Remind the adolescent to keep track of what happens for his or her "Test It Out" activity in the coming week.

"Okay, so it sounds like improving your friendships is very important to you and would likely help improve your mood and increase your activation. Is it SMART?"

- Go through each part of SMART and work with the teen to adjust the goal.
- Once a SMART goal has been identified, guide the adolescent through identifying mini-steps he or she can start with to ultimately accomplish his or her goal.
  - In breaking down tasks into their smallest possible steps—"mini-steps"—keep in mind that the first few steps should be relatively easy to accomplish, as this fosters success.
  - It is important to remember that we are working on encouraging and shaping new behavior patterns in adolescents who may be reluctant to try new things, so you may have to focus on small initial steps.
  - Use the "experiment" model to encourage the adolescent to identify things he or she can try to do and report back on.

"Nice job—so, your goal this week is to increase the amount of time you spend reaching out to your three closest friends, including spending 15 minutes each day engaged in things like initiating communication through social media, texts, or phone calls to these friends. Okay, so let's use this Goal-Setting worksheet (Handout 23) to schedule and map out mini-steps and also to determine who might be able to help you. This worksheet will also be a good way for you to keep track of what happens so that we can talk about it next time."

Thanks and Next Steps

- Let the adolescent know that you will briefly meet with their parent(s) to provide some information about how to support you.
- Assure the adolescent that issues that have come up in your meeting will not be discussed, unless he or she requests that they do.
- Preview that next module will focus on barriers to achieving goals.

▬▬▬▬▬▬▬▬▬▬ **PARENT(S) ONLY** ▬▬▬▬▬▬▬▬▬▬

"Welcome back! Today I wanted to touch base about a few things. Last time we focused on strategies to communicate with and support your teen—I'm curious to hear about what situations went well in addition to situations that didn't go so well. We will also talk about how you can continue to support your adolescent."

Ask the parent(s) whether they have any questions regarding the "Test It Out" activity: Handout 19 ("Communicating with Support: What Can You Do to Help an Interaction Go Well?") and answer any questions they might have. Discuss any challenges to completing the activity. Explore what the two experiences were like and identify whether it revealed an area in which it would be helpful for the parent to work or focus on with regard to supporting their adolescent.

Key Concept for Today's Session

Concept 1: Providing and Monitoring Support

*"Breaking the vicious cycle of depression is hard. As such, we feel that your adolescent will need support from you. Within the context of the BA model, this can mean many different things. For example, because the focus of treatment is on 'getting active' in all aspects of his or her life (e.g., physically, socially, academically, and within the family), it may mean, for example, offering your adolescent a ride to an activity at a time that is not completely convenient to you. Let's talk about effective ways for you to recognize what might be supportive, as well as techniques that will help you increase your level of support for your son or daughter. Giving support is different from helping or actually solving the problem. There are a lot of ways you can support your adolescent. Although there are a lot of different ways to support your son or daughter, the trick really lies in listening to your adolescent to figure out what will be supportive to him or her. These behaviors can be hard to identify—especially when your adolescent is really struggling and/or does not clearly let you know. Let's think about **what** behavior to support, then **how** to best support it."*

Introduce Handout 24 (Teaching Guide): "Ways to Support My Adolescent"

- Using Handout 24 ("Ways to Support My Adolescent"), brainstorm with the parent(s) ways they can support their adolescent by identifying as many specific supportive behaviors that they can think of and try.

- Be sure to praise the parents' creativity, pointing out their strengths and promoting their ownership of the ideas.

"You may have noticed that this list of supportive behaviors shows a number of things that you are already doing. I think the nice thing is that it is a good reminder that there are a number of simple things we can do to support adolescents who are struggling with depression and other issues. Sometimes it is easy to lose sight of how many

opportunities there are to be positive and supportive and how much our positive attention can be helpful and useful."

Introduce Handout 25 (Test It Out): "Monitoring Support"

"This week, I am going to ask you to complete a 'Test It Out' activity that relates to identifying and monitoring your supportive behaviors toward your adolescent.

"The bottom line is that monitoring our own supportive behaviors can actually help us be more supportive. Although you have already shared some excellent examples of how you support your adolescent, it should be a valuable tool in helping you turn up the intensity and frequency of your supportive behaviors, particularly as they relate to the goal of 'getting active.'"

Using Handout 25 ("Monitoring Support"), highlight that when we monitor the support we offer, it often gives us a better idea of where we might want to deliver more support. Emphasize that research suggests the following:

- Monitoring behaviors is an important step toward making successful behavior changes.
- The best way to monitor is to rate behaviors regularly.
- Monitoring support helps to:
  - Identify areas for personal growth.
  - Recognize current trends and progress.
  - Celebrate successes.
  - Prevent slips and slides.

Using Handout 25, help the parent(s) identify constructive support behaviors and ask them to track them over the next week.

Thanks and Next Steps

Thank the parent(s) for their participation today and ask whether there are further questions you can answer at this time. Preview that the next module will continue the discussion of how specifically to support their adolescent.

SESSION 7

Identifying Barriers

Suggested Total Session Time: 50–60 minutes

Session Overview

Goals

Session 7 centers on identifying barriers to accomplishing goals. Goals of this session are as follows:

1. Help the adolescent identify and overcome his or her barriers to accomplishing goals.
2. Practice by setting new goal(s) and identifying the mini-steps to get there.
3. Help the parent(s) support their adolescent.

Structure and Teaching Points

This session is structured to include a working session with the adolescent, followed by a joint session with the adolescent and parent(s) to discuss the ways in which the parent(s) can support their adolescent. Introduce the following core teaching concepts:

- It is important to recognize that there are often barriers to achieving goals.
  - Barriers can come from an external source, such as not having access to needed materials to accomplish a task or being prevented from completing a task by another person.
  - Barriers can also come from internal sources, such as not feeling like doing the task, getting distracted with other activities and so forth.
- Adolescents may need help overcoming barriers.
  - It is important to determine specific ways that the parent(s) can be helpful in overcoming barriers to specific goals (e.g., provide transportation to sporting events).
  - It is also important to discuss ways in which the parent(s) may create barriers to achieving goals.
- Transition to working with the parent(s) and adolescent together to address how the parent(s) can be supportive and help the adolescent.

Session Agenda

Adolescent Only

- Check-In
- Key Concepts for today's session:
  - Concept 1: How to Recognize and Get Around Barriers to Achieving Your Goal
    - Handout 26 (Teaching Guide): "Barriers: Internal versus External"
    - Handout 7 (Teaching Guide): "Getting Active!"
  - Concept 2: Setting a New Goal and Identifying the Mini-Steps to Get There
- "Test It Out" activity for the week: Handout 27 (Test It Out): "Goals and Barriers"

Adolescent and Parent(s) Together

- Review Handout 25 (Test It Out): "Monitoring Support"
- Key Concept for today's session:
  - Concept 1: Optimizing Support
    - Handout 28 (Teaching Guide): "Support Ideas"
    - Handout 29 (Test It Out): "Support Experiment"

Materials You Need to Have Ready:

- Today's Agenda
- SMFQ/PHQ-9
- Handout 23 (Test It Out): "Goal Setting"
- Handout 25 (Test It Out): "Monitoring Support"

- Handout 26 (Teaching Guide): "Barriers: Internal versus External"
- Handout 7 (Teaching Guide): "Getting Active!"
- Handout 27 (Test It Out): "Goals and Barriers"
- Handout 28 (Teaching Guide): "Support Ideas"
- Handout 29 (Test It Out): "Support Experiment"

Outline of Session

ADOLESCENT ONLY

Check-In

- Complete the SMFQ/PHQ-9.
- Review the SMFQ/PHQ-9.
- Generate Today's Agenda, including the allocation of time to review session material, as well as the Adolescent's Agenda items.

"Test It Out" Review: Handout 23: "Goal Setting"

- Review/complete Handout 23 ("Goal Setting") and determine how it worked for the adolescent to do the mini-steps and work toward his or her goal.
- Keep in mind the following types of questions:
  - *"Did you notice any change in your mood as you were taking these steps?"*
  - *"If you didn't notice any change in your mood, was there any sense of relief or accomplishment in getting any of your steps done?"*
  - *"Did anything get in the way of accomplishing your mini-steps?"*

Key Concepts for Today's Session

"The rationale for today's session is to discuss how we can identify barriers to our goals and find ways to overcome them, making it easier to accomplish the goal in the end. Every day there are goals that are either imposed upon us (get adolescent's example) or chosen by us (ask adolescent for another example). Nobody completes goals 100% of the time. It is essential to understand what gets in the way of completing goals. When something gets in the way of completing goals, we call it a 'barrier.'"

Using either last week's "Test It Out" or a situation that the adolescent can describe when he or she planned to complete a goal but did not, identify the barrier(s).

Concept 1: How to Recognize and Get Around Barriers to Achieving Your Goal

"Barriers can come from us as individuals or may result from something outside of ourselves, or outside of our control. We need to differentiate between 'internal' and 'external' barriers in order to help figure out the best ways to try to overcome them."

Introduce Handout 26 (Teaching Guide): "Barriers: Internal versus External"

"Internal barriers are things that are 'inside of us'—our thoughts, our feelings, our choices, and our behaviors—that prevent us from completing our goals. Examples of internal barriers might include things such as the following:

- Not feeling like it.
- Getting distracted by something that seemed more fun or interesting at the time.
- Ruminating or worrying so much about something that we never get around to it.
- Talking ourselves out of it.

"External barriers are things that are 'outside of us'—situations and events that prevent us from achieving our goals. These might be things such as the following:

- Not having all the necessary tools—for example, planning to attend gym class but noticing a big rip in your gym shorts.
- Not having the necessary support—for example, a friend who was supposed to come over and bring a laptop to begin a project called and canceled. Another example is planning to go to a movie but not having enough money."

Reintroduce Handout 7 (Teaching Guide): "Getting Active!"

Using Handout 7, highlight that one type of internal barrier has to do with acting according to a mood (mood-directed behavior), for example, "not feeling like it."

"Remember Session 3, in which we talked about mood-directed behavior and how our mood, feeling down or unmotivated, for example, can be an internally generated barrier to completing a goal.

"Today we want to talk more about the idea of using goal-directed, not mood-directed, behavior in such situations. In one of our earlier meetings, we talked about 'pump you up' activities—doing something you like even when you are feeling bad. Remember, we call that engaging in goal-directed behavior—that is, doing something positive even when we are feeling down as a way to get ourselves active and improve our mood. It is the idea that we work toward a goal rather than allowing our mood to dictate our actions. Using goal-directed behavior is a great strategy when you get bogged down by an internal barrier. We also want to talk about what to do when you are stuck with an external barrier. Remember in Session 5 when we talked about COPE and Problem Solving when you get triggered by something? External barriers can serve as triggers and are often very frustrating— you are trying your best to do something and you are prevented from being able to do it. In such situations, it is a great time to use COPE and problem solve your way around it. As a reminder, when faced with an external barrier, you would CALM and CLARIFY, generate OPTIONS, PERFORM an option, and EVALUATE. To sum up, internal barriers lead us to goal-directed behavior and external barriers lead us to COPE."

- Referring back to the "Test It Out" activity from the last session: Handout 23 (Test It Out): "Goal Setting," ask the adolescent if there were barriers to achieving the goal. If so, were the barriers internal? Was this an example of mood-directed behavior? Was this an example of getting stuck and not knowing how to problem solve? If so, coach the adolescent to use the appropriate skill—goal-directed behavior or COPE.
- Use the goal that the adolescent set for last week to discuss acting toward a goal rather than letting moods dictate behavior.

"Okay, let's see if we can put all this information about goals and identifying barriers into something practical that pertains to your life."

Concept 2: Setting a New Goal and Identifying the Mini-Steps to Get There

"Let's start by identifying another goal for the upcoming week [or refine last week's goal]. Remember what we talked about in the last session with regard to goals? A good goal is SMART—specifically stated, measurable, appealing, realistic, and time-bound. It can also be broken down into mini-steps and accomplished over time. If you were to identify another goal to work on over the course of the next week, what would you choose? [Note: It is fine for the adolescent to expand on his or her previous goal or to choose a new one.]

"Now that you have decided on the goal of _____, we can identify mini-steps you can take to begin working on reaching this goal, as well as barriers that could get in the way of your goal. Again, please remember that your goals are a 'work in progress,' and we will work together to fine-tune them over time.

"Let's go over what you are going to practice over the week and make sure to talk about any questions/concerns you wanted to make sure we addressed today (e.g., the adolescent's agenda). Then, you and I will meet briefly with your parent(s) to talk about how they may be supportive of you. I am then going to meet briefly with your parent(s) to touch base and talk with them about the exercise they did over the week."

"Test It Out" for the Coming Week: Introduce Handout 27 (Test It Out): "Goals and Barriers"

"You will have two 'Test It Out' worksheets for the week. First, work through goals and barriers using Handout 27."

- Set a goal in one area (Use Handout 22: "Identifying a SMART Goal" from Session 6, if needed):
- Use the adolescent's identified goal.
- Relative to the adolescent's goal, walk him or her through completion of the Handout 27 (Test It Out): "Goals and Barriers"—helping him or her to make sure the goal specified is SMART and has clear mini-steps.

Thanks and Next Steps

Let the adolescent know that you will now briefly meet with him or her and his or her parent(s):

- Remind the adolescent that you have been working with his or her parent(s) about being a good listener and providing support.
- Assure the adolescent that issues that have come up in your meeting will not be discussed, unless he or she requests that they do.

Share that the brief meeting between the therapist, adolescent, and parents will cover the following points:

- Highlight that you will all have a discussion about support, and that you hope the adolescent will speak up about what he or she finds helpful.
- Similar to mini-steps, point out that parent(s) will be more successful if the adolescent's requests for support are realistic, specifically stated, and mutually desirable.
- Preview that the next session focuses on overcoming avoidance.

ADOLESCENT AND PARENT(S) TOGETHER

"Welcome back! Today I wanted to talk with all of you about support. Review the 'Test It Out' activity from last week: Handout 25 (Test It Out): Monitoring Support."

- Ask about any observations and lesson learned.
- Review what they can take forward and apply to their "Test It Out" activity for the week.

Key Concept for Today's Session

Concept 1: Optimizing Support

"Let's continue to discuss support. I want us to focus on determining how your parent can best support you."

Introduce Handout 28 (Teaching Guide): "Support Ideas"

Review with the parent(s) and the adolescent the ways in which parents often show support.

- Discuss various options on the list.
- Ask the adolescent what he or she finds helpful.
- Add options that the adolescent identifies to the list.

Introduce Handout 29 (Test It Out): "Support Experiment"

- Ask the parent(s) and adolescent to agree on something the parent(s) can try in the coming week.
- Ask the parent(s) to track and monitor their support behavior throughout the week.

Thanks and Next Steps

Thank the adolescent and the parent(s) for their participation and ask whether there are further questions you can answer at this time. Preview that the next session for the adolescent will focus on overcoming avoidance, while the focus of the next session for the parent(s) will be a discussion of their experience of supporting their adolescent.

SESSION 8

Overcoming Avoidance

Suggested Total Session Time: 50–60 minutes

Session Overview

Goals

Session 8 centers on overcoming avoidance. Goals of this session are as follows:

1. Teach the adolescent to recognize barriers to activation, particularly escape/avoidance behaviors that get him or her stuck.
2. Teach the adolescent the concept of using alternative coping strategies when he or she recognizes avoidance/escape behaviors.

Structure and Teaching Points

This session is structured to include a working session with the adolescent, followed by a brief check-in and review of the parent(s) support experiment. Introduce the following core teaching concepts:

- A goal in BA is to identify and modify avoidance behaviors that serve the purpose of helping the adolescent escape or avoid negative feelings and overwhelming tasks but keep him or her stuck in a negative cycle of depression.
- *Avoidance behavior* is any behavior that makes a person feel a sense of relief, pleasure, or satisfaction in the short run but has negative long-term consequences.

- Avoidance works, temporarily, by removing one from aversive situations or feelings; but avoidance behaviors do not help to improve life in the long run.
- Once the adolescent can identify that his or her behavior is serving as avoidance, he or she can implement alternative strategies to help move him- or herself forward.
- The TRAP/TRAC is a process in which events, feelings, people, and so forth, that trigger avoidance are identified and alternative coping strategies are introduced.
- Engage parent(s) in a review and discussion of their experience with the monitoring support (i.e., Handout 29: "Support Experiment").

Session Agenda

Adolescent Only

- Check-In
- Key Concepts for today's session:
  - Concept 1: Understanding Avoidance
    - Handout 30 (Teaching Guide): What Does Avoidance Look Like?
  - Concept 2: Recognizing that Avoidance Works
  - Concept 3: Teaching the TRAP/TRAC Acronyms for Overcoming Avoidance
    - Handout 31 (Worksheet/Test It Out): "Using TRAP-TRAC to Conquer Avoidance and Overcome the Downward Spiral"
- "Test It Out" Activity for the week: Handout 31 (Worksheet/Test It Out): "Using TRAP-TRAC to Conquer Avoidance and Overcome the Downward Spiral"

Parent(s) Only

- Review Handout 29 (Test It Out): "Support Experiment"
- Key Concept for today's session:
  - Concept 1: Plan for the Final Phase of Treatment

Materials You Need to Have Ready

- Today's Agenda
- SMFQ/PHQ-9
- Handout 27 (Test It Out): "Goals and Barriers"
- Handout 30 (Teaching Guide): "What Does Avoidance Look Like?"
- Handout 31 (Worksheet/Test It Out): "Using TRAP-TRAC to Conquer Avoidance and Overcome the Downward Spiral" (2 copies)
- Handout 29 (Test It Out): "Support Experiment"

Outline of Session

ADOLESCENT ONLY

Check-In

- Complete the SMFQ/PHQ-9.
- Review the SMFQ/PHQ-9.
- Generate Today's Agenda, including the allocation of time to review session material, as well as the Adolescent's Agenda items.

"Test It Out" Review: Handout 27 (Test It Out): "Goals and Barriers"

- Review/complete Handout 27 ("Goals and Barriers") and discuss barriers that hindered goal completion, including any anticipated barriers that were encountered and any actual barriers that were not anticipated.
- Discuss problems encountered and skills utilized to overcome barriers.

Key Concepts for Today's Session

"The goal for today's session is to understand a specific kind of internal barrier—avoidance, which frequently gets in the way of getting things done. Understanding avoidance is important because it frequently feels good in the short run and gets us in trouble in the long run. . . ."

To illustrate this idea, use an example from the adolescent's life, if possible, to talk about briefly.

Concept 1: Understanding Avoidance

Introduce Handout 30 (Teaching Guide): "What Does Avoidance Look Like?"

"Avoidance is any behavior that makes us feel a sense of relief, pleasure, satisfaction, and so forth, in the short run, or that prolongs distress by allowing us to put off tasks we do not want to do. Avoidance can take a lot of different forms:

- *Procrastinating is a common and obvious form of avoidance. The interesting thing about procrastination is that it allows us to distract ourselves from the things we need to do, but unlike other forms of avoidance, it usually feels bad to procrastinate, even in the short run.*
- *Sometimes avoidance takes the form of brooding or thinking on and on about a problem—worrying it to death—without coming to any solution.*
- *A different form of avoidance is 'bursting,' or blowing up at people or situations and having a strong emotional reaction. This can get people off your back and get*

you out of doing an annoying task in the short run. However, it makes problems worse in the long run.
- A very common form of avoidance is just to 'shut down'; we can call this 'hibernating.' Staying in bed all day, not eating, avoiding friends, napping, and neglecting schoolwork all may be forms of hibernating. Do any of these resonate with you?"

Concept 2: Recognizing That Avoidance Works

"The thing about avoidance is that it works—**in the short run** there can be an immediate payoff, **but in the long run** there is a price! You can postpone activities that are a pain simply by avoiding and ignoring them. For example, you can wait until the night before a project is due to start it. Similarly, when you are feeling down or sad, it is easy to escape a miserable world through sleep. Although this might feel like the right or only thing to do in the moment, there is a long-term price. While avoidance works in the short run, in the long run it can make problems more stressful and contribute to a downward spiral."

- Overcoming avoidance is one of the main goals of BA, and it is one of the most important concepts the adolescent will learn.
- Help the adolescent identify an example of avoidance (or mood-directed behavior) from the previous few days.
- If the adolescent has difficulty thinking of an example, offer the following examples of avoidance:
  ○ Surfing the Web on the computer when you are supposed to be loading the dishwasher and cleaning the kitchen counters.
  ○ Tuning out, looking away when someone in authority is talking.
  ○ Sleeping because you feel lonely or bored.

Concept 3: Teaching the TRAP/TRAC Acronyms for Overcoming Avoidance

- Once the therapist and adolescent have identified an instance of avoidance (or mood-directed behavior), explain that one way to recognize when we are using avoidance is to think about being in a **TRAP**.
- TRAP is an acronym for Trigger, Response, and Avoidance Pattern. It is an easy way for us to think about the function of avoidance.

Introduce Handout 31 (Worksheet): "Using TRAP-TRAC to Conquer Avoidance and Overcome the Downward Spiral"

*"Let's take your example and walk through how it became a **TRAP**:*

- *Trigger: What happened? For example: having a disagreement with a friend.*
- *Response: What did you feel or have the urge to do? For example, feeling sad and thinking, 'I don't want to deal with this'; wanting to be alone.*
- *Avoidance Pattern TRAP: What did you do to avoid feeling badly? What did you do to avoid doing something you really did not want to do? For example, not calling your friend, staying home so as not to see your friend.*

"When you have identified a TRAP, the objective is to get out of the trap and get back on TRAC.

*"The Trigger and Response are the same, but to get back on track you would figure out how to use **Alternative Coping** rather than getting into an **Avoidance Pattern**."*

- The therapist should use the TRAP-TRAC worksheet to demonstrate this concept to the adolescent.
    - Remind the adolescent that when he or she engages in avoidance, the adolescent is engaging in mood-directed behavior, but when he or she engages in alternative coping, the adolescent is engaging in goal-directed behavior.
    - Emphasize that getting out of avoidance patterns may not make him or her feel better right away.
    - Since we usually escape or avoid aversive feelings or situations, we may even feel a little worse when we use alternative coping rather than avoidance.
    - Think about this as developing a new habit. It will take time and practice—one try probably will not be enough.
    - If the old habit has been avoidance, the new habit is to recognize the trigger and response, and use alternative coping.

"There are several ways to break out of avoidance patterns and get started with alternative coping. Two possibilities that you already know how to do include the following:

- 1. *Identifying and practicing a mini-step toward a goal or activity, as we did in Sessions 6 and 7.*
    - Review: Identify a goal related to the situation that triggered avoidance, and take one mini-step toward that goal. For example:
        - The trigger was having an argument with a friend.
        - The ongoing goal is 'to be nicer to my friends.'

- *A mini-step might be sending a text to my friend, saying, 'Sorry I was grouchy.'*
- *If that is too hard, another mini-step would be to send a friendly text to someone else.*
- *Alternatively, you could identify a goal unrelated to the trigger situation, and complete a mini-step to keep you moving forward. For example, focus on a goal of learning to play the guitar, and take the mini-step of practicing some chords or a song."*

- 2. Using COPE problem solving, as in Session 5.
  - Review: There are four basic steps to problem solving:
    - Step 1: **CALM** and **CLARIFY**.
    - Step 2: Generate **OPTIONS**.
    - Step 3: **PERFORM**.
    - Step 4: **EVALUATE**.
- If the adolescent is having trouble remembering these concepts, the therapist can reintroduce Handouts 16 ("Using COPE") and 20 ("Setting SMART Goals").

"Test It Out" for the Coming Week: Use Handout 31 (Test It Out):
"Using TRAP-TRAC to Conquer Avoidance and Overcome the Downward Spiral"
(Second Copy)

"Your 'Test It Out' work for the week is to pay attention to a situation/trigger and your response using Handout 31. Identify whether you got stuck in the avoidance pattern or were able to use alternative coping; record what you did and rate how you felt."

Thanks and Next Steps

Let the adolescent know that you will now briefly meet with his or her parent(s) to review their experience with the "support experiment." Remind the adolescent that there are about four sessions left, and that we can use this time to think about and practice strategies that will work best to solve the adolescent's problems and improve mood.

▰▰▰ PARENT(S) ONLY ▰▰▰

Review Handout 29 (Test It Out): "Support Experiment"

"Welcome back! Today I wanted to talk with you about your experience with the Support Experiment (Handout 29).

Review the "Test It Out" activity from last week: Handout 29 (Test It Out): "Support Experiment."

- Review with parent(s) their experience of trying to provide support, using Handout 29 from the previous week. Ask about barriers.
- Review what the parent(s) can take forward.
- Ask parents to continue to work on providing support to their adolescent's efforts to manage his or her moods and activities.

Key Concept for Today's Session

Concept 1: Plan for the Final Phase of Treatment

- Discuss end-of-treatment goals.
- Structure/focus of remaining sessions:
  - Remind the parent(s) that four sessions are left and in the next three sessions the focus is on helping the adolescent to put his or her skills into practice in ways that will continue to help manage his or her moods and activities. Let them know that we do not plan to meet with them as part of these sessions, but they can let us know if they need some time or have something they need to bring up.
  - Review with the parent(s) whether there are specific concerns/issues that they hope could be integrated into work of the next sessions—reminding them that the focus is on reducing the adolescent's depression.
  - Let them know that in the final session we will develop a plan to help their adolescent to stay on track.

Thanks and Next Steps

Thank the parent(s) for their participation today and ask whether there are further questions you can answer at this time. Preview that the next sessions will focus on review of concepts the adolescent has learned throughout treatment and will be geared more to the individual needs of their adolescent.

MODULE 4

Practice

SESSION 9

Putting It All Together

Suggested Total Session Time: 50–60 minutes

Session Overview

Goals

Session 9 centers on working with the adolescent to identify the areas of their greatest need. Goals of this session are as follows:

1. Review with the adolescent where he or she is in terms of his or her depression, as well as other important variables in the adolescent's life (e.g., conflict with sibling, sleep), making connections among situations, activities, and moods.
2. Help the adolescent identify what he or she wants to focus on for the remaining treatment sessions.
3. Review key skills that might be important in helping the adolescent work toward his or her goal.

Structure and Teaching Points

This session is structured to include a review of previous material with the adolescent and discussion of how BA can be used to move the adolescent toward his or her goals. Introduce the following core teaching concepts/points:

- Highlight connections between situations and behaviors associated with changes in the adolescent's mood and functioning based on patterns observed over the course of treatment.
- Stress the importance of selecting and tailoring skills learned in treatment to his or her individual needs and experiences.
- Review the range of skills covered in BA, including getting active, making the most out of good moments, COPE, setting goals, recognizing barriers, and overcoming avoidance.

Session Agenda

Adolescent Only

- Check-In
- Key Concept for today's session:
  - Concept 1: Taking Stock
    - Handout 32 (Worksheet): "Taking Stock"
    - Handout 33 (Worksheet): "Developing an Action Plan"
    - Handout 34 (Worksheet/Test It Out): "Action Plan"
- "Test It Out" activity for the week: Handout 34 (Test It Out): "Action Plan"

Materials You Need to Have Ready

- Today's Agenda
- SMFQ/PHQ-9
- Handout 31 (Test It Out): "Using TRAP-TRAC to Conquer Avoidance and Overcome the Downward Spiral"
- Handout 32 (Worksheet): "Taking Stock"
- Handout 33 (Worksheet): "Developing an Action Plan"
- Handout 2 (Worksheet): "How Behavioral Activation Works for You"
- Handout 34 (Test It Out): "Action Plan"
- Handout 27 (Test It Out): "Goals and Barriers"
- Have ready access to teaching guides and worksheets from prior sessions to draw on as needed.

Outline of Session

ADOLESCENT ONLY

Check-In

- Complete the SMFQ/PHQ-9.
- Review the SMFQ/PHQ-9.
- Generate Today's Agenda, including the allocation of time to review session material, as well as the Adolescent's Agenda items.

"Test It Out" Review: Handout 31 (Test It Out): "Using TRAP-TRAC to Conquer Avoidance and Overcome the Downward Spiral"

- Review/complete identification of an avoidance pattern and what the adolescent has used/could use for alternative coping.
- Discuss problems encountered, troubleshooting barriers to use of alternative coping strategies, and identifying alternative coping strategies if needed.

Key Concept for Today's Session

"Today we are going to look back over how things have gone for you since you began therapy: what your life was like before, how your life is now, and what you would like your life to be like as you move forward. This will help us set priorities about what to focus on for the next few therapy sessions."

Concept 1: Taking Stock

Introduce Handout 32 (Worksheet): "Taking Stock"

"You now have been coming to therapy for several weeks. As we begin to think about wrapping up our time together over the next several sessions, it is often helpful to take a look back with regard to where you have been, take a look at the present, get a good assessment of where you are now, and project into the future and talk about where you want to go. We call this 'Taking Stock.'"

Use Handout 32 ("Taking Stock") to review with the adolescent how his or her mood ratings have changed over time, as well as changes in other areas, and challenges or goals on which he or she has worked in therapy so far. Revisit Handout 2 ("How Behavioral Activation Works for You") from Session 1 to review what was going on when the adolescent started therapy, changes he or she has made, and so forth. Some adolescents find it helpful to consult weekly symptom ratings, including plotting them on the timeline, whereas others are able to reflect on the timing and map it out without integrating all of the specific data.

Setting Goals/Priorities

- Remind the adolescent of how many sessions remain.
- Let the adolescent know that the focus today is to work on developing a plan for the use of the remaining therapy sessions, as well as to begin developing a plan to stay on a positive track.
- Help the adolescent identify what he or she wants to focus on by reviewing areas in which he or she has made significant gains and areas that may still need some practice and work.
- Translate all this into a goal that is SMART (feel free to pull in Handout 27: "Goals and Barriers," if it is helpful to the adolescent in setting and monitoring a goal).
- Work with the adolescent to identify what steps he or she wants to try over the next week, then help him or her to identify barriers that might get in the way.
- Review key skills that might be important in helping the adolescent work toward his or her goal—ways to get active, make the most of good moments, using COPE, goal setting, identifying barriers, and overcoming avoidance.

"Test It Out" for the Coming Week: Introduce Handout 34 (Test It Out): "Action Plan"

- The "Test It Out" activity will need to be individualized for each adolescent. Use Handout 34 ("Action Plan") for Session 9 and beyond as one tool to help the youth identify goals, set priorities, and outline activities and skills that will ultimately help him or her in moving forward. The "Action Plan" is a tool to define the big picture and can be modified over time. Because it remains important to track progress, the therapist should discuss this with each adolescent, utilizing tools that he or she finds specifically helpful (e.g., phone, computer, school planner).
- Help the adolescent develop a specific (what, when, where, with whom) plan regarding positive activities in which he or she will engage, as well as specific ways he or she can reward him- or herself for the things attempted/worked on.

Thanks and Next Steps

"Let's go over what you are going to practice over the week and make sure to talk about any questions/concerns that you want to make sure we addressed today (e.g., the Adolescent's Agenda)."

Preview that the next module will focus on more individualized practice.

SESSIONS 10 AND 11

Practicing Skills

Suggested Total Session Time: 50–60 minutes

Session Overview

The therapist should use this section of Module 4 flexibly. While it was designed to last for two sessions (Sessions 10 and 11), more individualized practice may be needed and it could extend for three or more sessions, whatever is appropriate to the adolescent and his or her situation.

Goals

Sessions 10 and 11 center on working with the adolescent to identify the areas of his or her greatest need. Goals of these sessions are as follows:

1. Identify areas of greatest need and challenge.
2. Support the adolescent as he or she uses the skills presented in earlier sessions to move toward his or her goal(s) and overcome barriers in goal achievement.
3. Review the importance of maintaining a focus on working to improve mood/depression. The focus of the work should be on strategies that will help the adolescent with mood management—this may be schoolwork or strategies to manage parental demands—but it should always come back to the application and practice of core BA principles.

Structure and Teaching Points

Sessions 10 and 11 are structured to include a review of previous material with the adolescent and discussion of how he or she can use BA to move toward his or her goals. Introduce the following core teaching concept(s):

- Review the adolescent's customized Action Plan to highlight the use of BA skills over the course of the past week and to discuss progress and challenges.
- Review the range of skills covered in behavioral activation, which includes getting active, making the most of good feelings, using COPE, goal setting, identifying barriers, and overcoming avoidance.
- Consider how to help the adolescent develop his or her Action Plan to keep moving forward, including how he or she will handle setbacks.

Session Agenda

Adolescent Only

- Check-In
- Key Concept for today's session:
  - Concept 1: Review
    - Handout 34 (Test It Out): "Action Plan"
- "Test It Out" Activity for the week: Handout 34 (Test It Out): "Action Plan"

Materials You Need to Have Ready

- Today's Agenda
- SMFQ/PHQ-9
- Handout 34 (Test It Out): "Action Plan"
- Have ready access to teaching guides and worksheets from prior sessions to draw on as needed.

Outline of Session

ADOLESCENT ONLY

Check-In

- Complete the SMFQ/PHQ-9.
- Review the SMFQ/PHQ-9.
- Generate Today's Agenda, including the allocation of time to review session material, as well as the Adolescent's Agenda items.

"Test It Out" Activity from Last Week: Review Handout 34: "Action Plan"

Review/complete worksheet and praise the adolescent for his or her effort/success, or troubleshoot barriers if the adolescent was unable to engage in alternative coping.

Key Concept for Today's Session

"As we begin to wrap up our time together and start thinking about you going out and trying this all on your own, we not only want to think about your goals and priorities moving forward, but also to spend some time reviewing all the different skills we have talked about, which ones have worked well, and which might need some more practice."

Concept 1: Review

Use the adolescent's Action Plan developed last week to guide a discussion about what he or she did last week and his or her plan will be for the coming week. Focus the discussion on what worked well and what barriers the adolescent faced, including a discussion of issues related to avoidance. Tweak the plan as needed and include a review of skills that the adolescent could have employed in challenging situations but perhaps forgot about or struggled to apply effectively. Based on the discussion and what you know about the adolescent historically, anticipate barriers with the adolescent and proactively review strategies to overcome them. Be sure to pull forward any needed teaching guides from previous sessions.

"Test It Out" for the Coming Week: Introduce Handout 34 (Test It Out): "Action Plan"

"This week, the 'Test It Out' activity is an extension of the work you did last week. We want to continue to tweak your Action Plan over the next couple of weeks. As we talked about previously, we are in a phase of treatment in which we just want to keep practicing skills, applying them in challenging situations, then coming back together to talk about how it went. Let's go over what you are going to practice this week and also make sure that we have talked about any other questions/concerns you might have at this point [e.g., the Adolescent's Agenda]."

- Continue to use the adolescent's Action Plan and the activities and strategies specified for the coming week. You can build on the adolescent's Action Plan from last week, or you can start a new one depending on how the session went and the focus of the work.
- Since the plan will vary from adolescent to adolescent, the therapist needs to note carefully (i.e., make a copy) the agreed-upon "Test It Out" activity.

Thanks and Next Steps

- Session 10: Review the number of remaining sessions and highlight that the next session will continue to focus on refining the adolescent's Action Plan, with a goal of moving forward and coping with setbacks.

- Session 11 or the point at which the adolescent moves toward termination: Preview that the next module will focus on a relapse prevention and termination.

MODULE 5
Moving Forward

SESSION 12

Relapse Prevention and Saying Good-Bye

Suggested Total Session Time: 50–60 minutes

Session Overview

The therapist should use Module 5 flexibly. While it was designed to last one session (Session 12), it is recognized that every adolescent is unique, and termination and relapse prevention may require more time in some cases.

Goals

This session marks the end of treatment and involves a discussion of relapse prevention, specifically focusing on the adolescent's challenges and strengths, and how to recognize and manage those challenges moving forward. Goals of this session are as follows:

1. Work with the adolescent to identify challenges moving forward (e.g., vulnerability to depressive symptoms in the face of certain situations, triggers, and transitions).
2. Discuss the difference in the adolescent's response to those challenges before and after treatment, specifically identifying skills that have been used to help the adolescent feel better and prevent a downward spiral and the vicious cycle of depression.

3. Develop a relapse prevention plan that outlines the adolescent's identified triggers and strategies he or she can use to avoid spiraling down into depression, drawing on the skills presented over the course of therapy.
4. With the adolescent and parent(s) together, discuss thoughts and ideas about how they would know when additional treatment might be useful.

Structure and Teaching Points

This module is structured to include a working session with the adolescent, followed by a brief check-in with the parent(s) and adolescent together. Introduce the following core teaching concepts:

- Slips are common and natural and a sign for the adolescent to take action in order to keep moving forward.
- It is best to be prepared for slips by developing a Relapse Prevention Plan that includes thinking through triggers, signs of slipping, and coping skills and strategies to manage.
- Others, such as the parent(s) or other trusted adults, can support the adolescent with managing slips and maintaining his or her "Doing What Works" (Handout 35) and "Action Plan" (Handout 34) moving forward.
- Engage the parent(s) and adolescent together, allowing time to address parent(s) questions and concerns, and engage them in reviewing the Relapse Prevention Plan, "Doing What Works" (Handout 35), and the "Action Plan" (Handout 34) for moving forward.

Session Agenda

Adolescent Only

- Check-In
- Key Concepts for today's session:
  - Concept 1: What Is a "Slip"?
  - Concept 2: Doing What Works
    - Handout 35 (Worksheet): "Doing What Works"

Adolescent and Parent(s) Together

- Key Concept for today's session:
  - Concept 1: Review Relape Prevention Plan and Action Plan
    - Review Handout 35 (Worksheet): "Doing What Works"
    - Handout 34 (Worksheet): "Action Plan"

Materials You Need to Have Ready

- Today's Agenda
- SMFQ/PHQ-9
- Handout 34 (Worksheet/Test It Out): "Action Plan"
- Handout 35 (Worksheet): "Doing What Works"

Outline of Session

ADOLESCENT ONLY

Check-In

- Complete the SMFQ/PHQ-9.
- Review the SMFQ/PHQ-9.
- Generate Today's Agenda, including the allocation of time to review session material, as well as the Adolescent's Agenda items.

"Test It Out" Review: Handout 34 (Worksheet/Test It Out): "Action Plan"

- Review/complete the handout and praise the adolescent's effort/success, or troubleshoot barriers with him or her if he or she was unable to engage in the alternative coping.
- Discuss problems encountered and skills utilized to overcome barriers.

Key Concepts for Today's Session

"Since this is our last session, I want to take some time to review what you have accomplished over the last 3 months and to thank you for all your hard work. I would also like to work with you to think ahead about what kinds of pitfalls you might run into and what you can do to prevent or reverse a downward spiral that could lead to feeling depressed again. Today we'll take everything you learned and talk about what works for you."

Concept 1: What Is a "Slip"?

"Slips are common; it's natural to feel badly when crummy things happen. One way to think about it is that a SLIP is like tripping on the stairs. Usually we just slip, which is only one step down the staircase—then we can quickly get going up the stairs again. SLIPS can be scary, but they do not have to lead to plunging down the stairs. To keep moving forward—with all the good work you have been doing, it's helpful to think a bit about what you will do if you slip now and then. The bottom line is that a slip is a sign to take action in order to keep moving forward."

Concept 2: Doing What Works

Introduce Handout 35 (Worksheet): "Doing What Works"

"As you know, new challenges are going to come up. Let's take some time not only to think through and highlight those challenges but to also consider strategies that have worked for you in the past. Let's reflect on the last few months and identify triggers, signs of slipping, skills that have worked, and who can support you."

- Step through the list of potential triggers with the adolescent. Encourage him or her to reflect on past triggers, as well as likely upcoming triggers such as transitioning to high school or college, experiencing a breakup, or ongoing tension or conflict with parents.
- Discuss signs of slipping, including feelings, body signs, and avoidant and risky behaviors.
- Reflect on coping skills that have worked in the past, reviewing things such as goal setting, making the most of good moments, evaluating the payoff and price of behavior, using COPE, planning "Pump You Up" activities, recognizing TRAPs, and getting back on TRAC.
- Discuss the adolescent's supports and who can help him or her.

"Test It Out" for the Coming Week: Review Handout 34 (Test It Out): "Action Plan"

"Even though we are winding down our therapy together, continuing to work toward your goals is essential. So our final 'Test It Out' activity is an extension of the work you have been doing the last few weeks. I want you to continue to tweak your Action Plan and keep working on moving toward your goals. Let's take a minute to talk through what you are going to practice this week and how you can keep this process going."

- Build on the adolescent's Action Plan from last week, or start a new one depending on how the session went and the focus of the work.
- Work with the adolescent to think "What next?" in terms of his or her goals, and ministeps. Help him or her think about how to continue to develop and refine Action Plans as he or she moves forward.

Thanks and Next Steps

Let the adolescent know that you will now briefly meet with him or her and his or her parent(s) to cover the following points:

- Let the adolescent know that together you will review the Relapse Prevention Plan and the Action Plan.
- Encourage the adolescent to take an active role in presenting these plans to his or her parent(s).

ADOLESCENT AND PARENT(S) TOGETHER

"Welcome back! Today we want to talk with you about your child's progress and plans moving forward."

Key Concept for Today's Session

Concept 1: Review Relapse Prevention Plan and Action Plan

- Discuss the likelihood of "slips" (see earlier discussion).
- Introduce Handout 35 (Worksheet): "Doing What Works"
  - Have the adolescent walk through the worksheet and encourage his or her parent(s) to add their perspective and ideas.
  - Discuss what the adolescent and parent(s) might look for that would suggest more than a slip but a return of significant depressive symptoms indicating that returning to treatment would be helpful.
- Introduce Handout 34 (Worksheet/Test It Out): "Action Plan"
  - If the adolescent is willing to share his or her Action Plan with the parent(s), encourage him/her to do so. Otherwise, review the overall plan, including the specific skills that he or she plans to use.

Thanks and Appreciation

Thank the adolescent and his or her parent(s) for their participation and ask whether there are further questions you can answer at this time.

Saying Good-Bye

Highlight how the adolescent and his or her parent(s) can communicate with you should they need support in the future.

Reproducible Handouts

Handout 1	Behavioral Activation Model	175
Handout 2	How Behavioral Activation Works for You	176
Handout 3	Activity Monitoring	177
Handout 4	Who and What Is on "First" in Your Life?	178
Handout 5	Downward Spiral, Upward Spiral	179
Handout 6	A Parent Guide to Adolescent Depression	180
Handout 7	Getting Active!	183
Handout 8	Activity–Mood Chart—Example	184
Handout 9	Activity–Mood Chart	185
Handout 10	Ways to Describe Parenting an Adolescent	186
Handout 11	Short- versus Long-Term Consequences	187
Handout 12	Pump You Up, Bring You Down	188
Handout 13	Activities Menu	189
Handout 14	Activities That Help to PUMP You UP!!	190
Handout 15	Using COPE to Solve Problems	191
Handout 16	Using COPE	192
Handout 17	How to Communicate with Support	193

Handout 18	Practicing How to Communicate with Support	194
Handout 19	Communicating with Support: What Can You Do to Help an Interaction Go Well?	195
Handout 20	Setting SMART Goals	196
Handout 21	How SMART Is This Goal?	197
Handout 22	Identifying a SMART Goal	198
Handout 23	Goal Setting	199
Handout 24	Ways to Support My Adolescent	200
Handout 25	Monitoring Support	201
Handout 26	Barriers: Internal versus External	202
Handout 27	Goals and Barriers	203
Handout 28	Support Ideas	204
Handout 29	Support Experiment	205
Handout 30	What Does Avoidance Look Like?	206
Handout 31	Using TRAP-TRAC to Conquer Avoidance and Overcome the Downward Spiral	207
Handout 32	Taking Stock	208
Handout 33	Developing an Action Plan	209
Handout 34	Action Plan	210
Handout 35	Doing What Works	211

HANDOUT 1

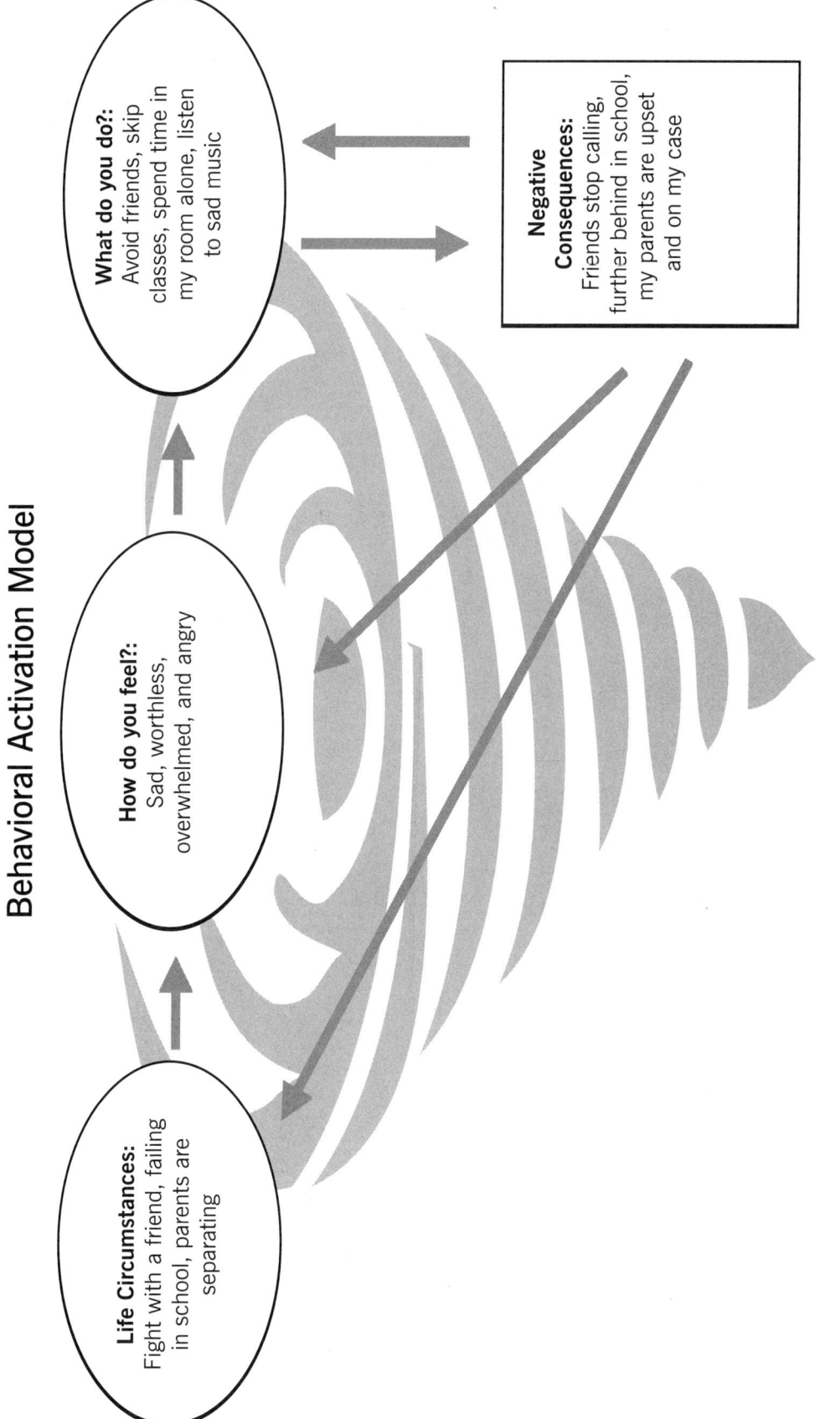

Behavioral Activation Model

Life Circumstances: Fight with a friend, failing in school, parents are separating

How do you feel?: Sad, worthless, overwhelmed, and angry

What do you do?: Avoid friends, skip classes, spend time in my room alone, listen to sad music

Negative Consequences: Friends stop calling, further behind in school, my parents are upset and on my case

From *Behavioral Activation with Adolescents: A Clinician's Guide* by Elizabeth McCauley, Kelly A. Schloredt, Gretchen R. Gudmundsen, Christopher R. Martell, and Sona Dimidjian. Copyright © 2016 The Guilford Press. Permission to photocopy this handout is granted to purchasers of this book for personal use or use with individual clients (see copyright page for details). Purchasers can download additional copies of this handout (see the box at the end of the table of contents).

HANDOUT 2

How Behavioral Activation Works for You

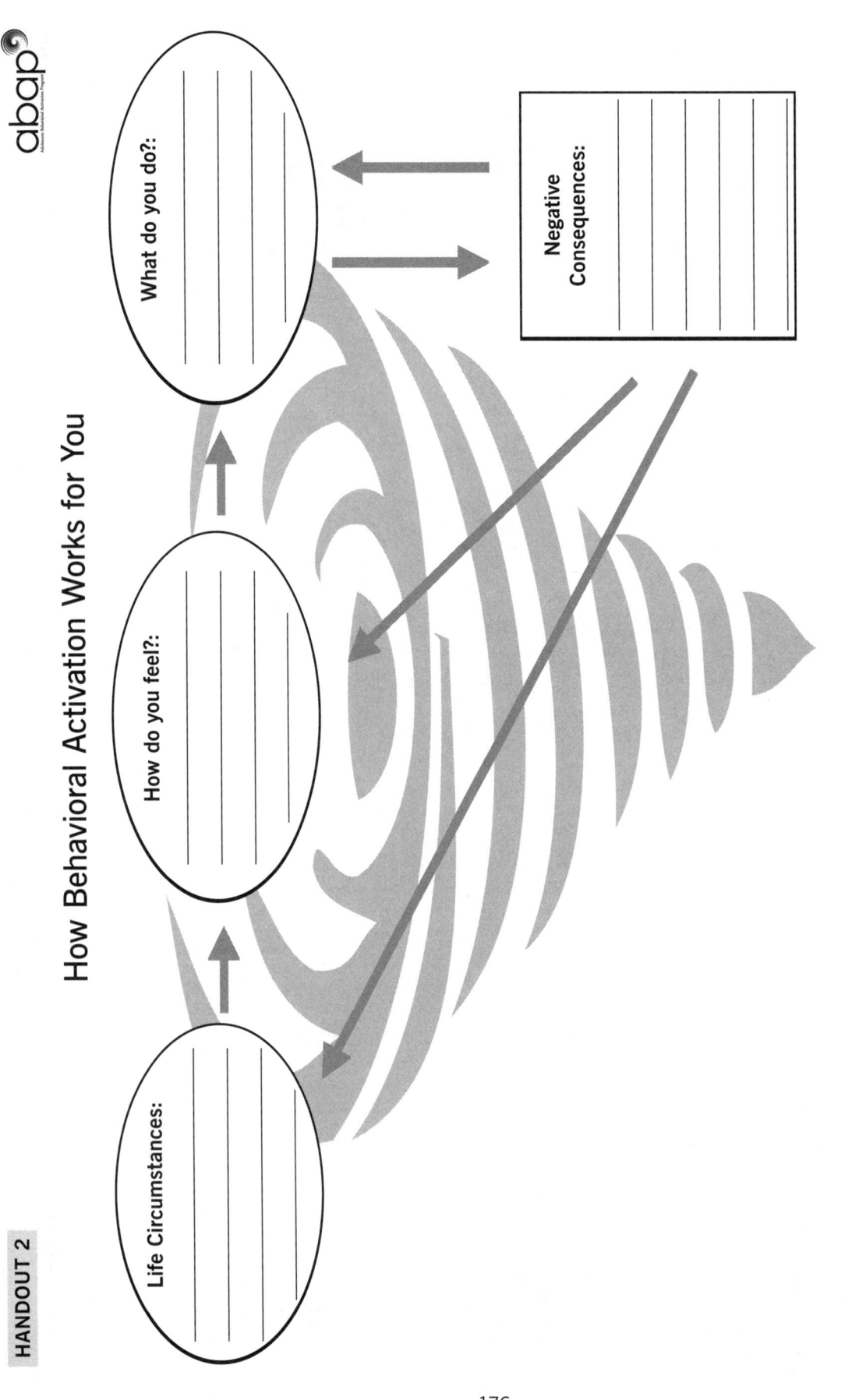

Life Circumstances:

How do you feel?:

What do you do?:

Negative Consequences:

From Behavioral Activation with Adolescents: A Clinician's Guide by Elizabeth McCauley, Kelly A. Schloredt, Gretchen R. Gudmundsen, Christopher R. Martell, and Sona Dimidjian. Copyright © 2016 The Guilford Press. Permission to photocopy this handout is granted to purchasers of this book for personal use or use with individual clients (see copyright page for details). Purchasers can download additional copies of this handout (see the box at the end of the table of contents).

HANDOUT 3

Activity Monitoring

Here's what to do:
- With your clinician, outline your activities for today (up to now), then complete the remainder at home tonight.
- Choose one other day this week and keep track of your activities.
- In each time slot, fill in what you were doing.

Date/Day:	Activity
7 AM	
8 AM	
9 AM	
10 AM	
11 AM	
NOON	
1 PM	
2 PM	
3 PM	
4 PM	
5 PM	
6 PM	
7 PM	
8 PM	
9 PM	
10 PM	
11 PM	
12+	

Date/Day:	Activity
7 AM	
8 AM	
9 AM	
10 AM	
11 AM	
NOON	
1 PM	
2 PM	
3 PM	
4 PM	
5 PM	
6 PM	
7 PM	
8 PM	
9 PM	
10 PM	
11 PM	
12+	

From *Behavioral Activation with Adolescents: A Clinician's Guide* by Elizabeth McCauley, Kelly A. Schloredt, Gretchen R. Gudmundsen, Christopher R. Martell, and Sona Dimidjian. Copyright © 2016 The Guilford Press. Permission to photocopy this handout is granted to purchasers of this book for personal use or use with individual clients (see copyright page for details). Purchasers can download additional copies of this handout (see the box at the end of the table of contents).

HANDOUT 4

Who and What Is on "First" in Your Life?

Think of your world—from your perspective, who are YOUR important people and what are YOUR important activities? What's most important? Identify which people and activities help you feel good. Are there people or activities that bring you down?

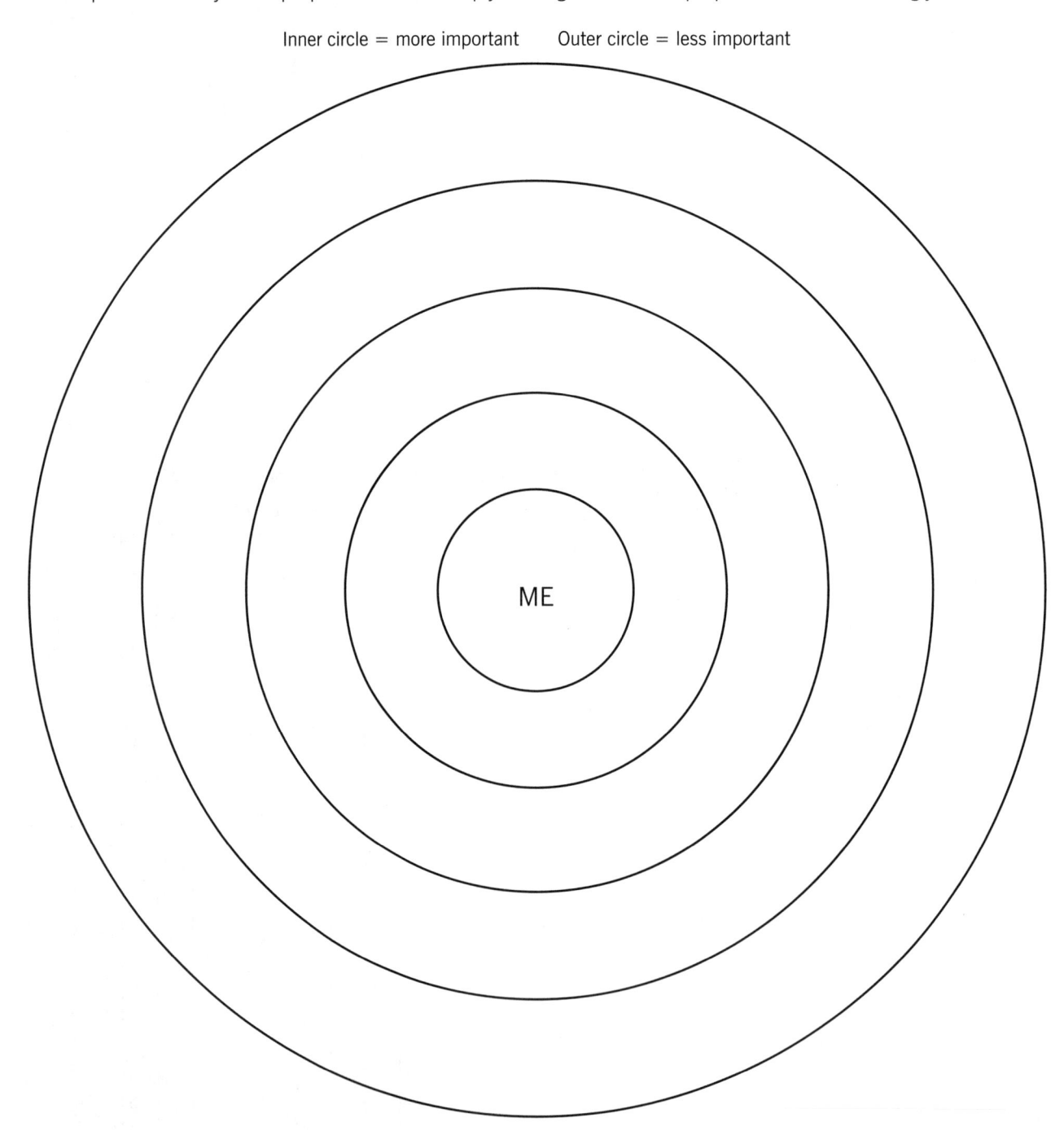

Inner circle = more important   Outer circle = less important

ME

From *Behavioral Activation with Adolescents: A Clinician's Guide* by Elizabeth McCauley, Kelly A. Schloredt, Gretchen R. Gudmundsen, Christopher R. Martell, and Sona Dimidjian. Copyright © 2016 The Guilford Press. Permission to photocopy this handout is granted to purchasers of this book for personal use or use with individual clients (see copyright page for details). Purchasers can download additional copies of this handout (see the box at the end of the table of contents).

HANDOUT 5

Downward Spiral, Upward Spiral

Keep track of one thing that happened over the week that brought your mood DOWN:

1. What happened?
   _____
   _____
   _____

2. How did you feel?
   _____
   _____

3. What did you do?
   _____
   _____

4. Did you feel better or worse?
   _____
   _____

Keep track of one thing that happened over the week that brought your mood UP:

1. What happened?
   _____
   _____
   _____

2. How did you feel?
   _____
   _____

3. What did you do?
   _____
   _____

4. Did you feel better or worse?
   _____
   _____

From *Behavioral Activation with Adolescents: A Clinician's Guide* by Elizabeth McCauley, Kelly A. Schloredt, Gretchen R. Gudmundsen, Christopher R. Martell, and Sona Dimidjian. Copyright © 2016 The Guilford Press. Permission to photocopy this handout is granted to purchasers of this book for personal use or use with individual clients (see copyright page for details). Purchasers can download additional copies of this handout (see the box at the end of the table of contents).

HANDOUT 6

A Parent Guide to Adolescent Depression

Depression is a problem that many adolescents face. For some it comes out of the blue; others have been trying to cope with feeling down and unmotivated for a long time. When he or she is depressed, you may notice a number of changes in your adolescent:

- feeling down or cranky and irritable
- feeling like things are no longer fun
- feeling tired and low energy
- finding it hard to concentrate and complete schoolwork
- feeling less interested in spending time with family and friends

Sometimes things might feel so bad that your adolescent may have a hard time imagining how things will ever be better.

Depression can be a "vicious cycle." It is often the case that the more depressed the adolescent feels, the less he or she wants to do, and the less he or she does, the more depressed he or she feels. Because of this vicious cycle, we find that depression often gets in the way of adolescents' participation in activities with friends and family and making progress in school.

Depression is just a signal that something in the adolescent's life needs to be changed. Many adolescents can identify "triggers" to their depression—an event or series of events that happened before they started feeling depressed. "Triggers" commonly related to depression include things such as having a fight with a friend or parent(s); a breakup; not making a team or club; losing something important; feeling overwhelmed by school; and having a hard time with peer relationships.

After such "triggers" or events "kick off" feelings of depression, it can be hard to figure out ways to feel better. Adolescents might isolate themselves, not want to be around family, hide out in their room or spend more and more time online, sleep a lot more or stay up late into the night, or avoid friends and activities. These behaviors can make depression worse, leading many adolescents and their parent(s) to seek help.

Coping with the Problem

There are different treatments for depressed teenagers. Some treatments involve taking medication and others involve "talk therapy." One type of "talk therapy" is behavioral activation therapy, in which adolescents work with their therapists to stop the "vicious cycle" of depression and figure out ways to reengage in the activities that are important to them. In order to do this, the adolescent works with the therapist to identify the triggers that are related to his or her feelings of sadness or loss of motivation and identify problems in his or her life that he or she would like to change. The therapist shares some skills or strategies that have been found to help overcome depression and supports the adolescent as he or she sets goals and fine-tunes strategies to help him or her cope with depression and make his or her life more fulfilling. The therapist supports the adolescent in taking steps to achieve his or her goals. Although it can require effort and hard work, the adolescent can break the "vicious cycle" of depression through guided activity.

(continued)

From *Behavioral Activation with Adolescents: A Clinician's Guide* by Elizabeth McCauley, Kelly A. Schloredt, Gretchen R. Gudmundsen, Christopher R. Martell, and Sona Dimidjian. Copyright © 2016 The Guilford Press. Permission to photocopy this handout is granted to purchasers of this book for personal use or use with individual clients (see copyright page for details). Purchasers can download additional copies of this handout (see the box at the end of the table of contents).

A Parent Guide to Adolescent Depression *(page 2 of 3)*

What Will the Therapist Do?

Sometimes it is hard to "just do it" and change behavior on your own. If changing behavior were really easy, none of us would ever need to ask for help—but most of us benefit from help when we are struggling with something difficult. When adolescents are learning new skills, such as algebra, basketball, knitting, or skiing, they often have a coach, a teacher, or a guide. Because behavioral activation therapy involves learning new skills and trying new activities, the therapist serves as a coach or guide. The therapist teaches new skills and coaches or guides the adolescent as he or she tries these new strategies out in real life and practices them. We call this *guided activity*. The activities in behavioral activation therapy are not the same for all adolescents. Your adolescent's therapist will work closely with him or her to figure out what activities are right for him or her, what activities will help decrease the depression, and what activities will help him or her feel more in control of life.

Why Focus on Getting Active?

There are many good reasons to become active, particularly for someone who is feeling depressed:

1. Guided activity can help improve mood. Even when depressed, being active can help a person feel in control of his or her life. Even when engaging in an activity that seems like a real drag, such as cleaning or doing homework, being active frequently brings with it a sense of accomplishment.
2. Guided activity can help a person feel less tired. Even though staying in bed or taking naps after school may seem like a good idea to a depressed adolescent, extra sleep is just another way to isolate. Guided activity, even when a person feels tired, can lead to feeling more energetic and spunky. For example, if your adolescent really likes playing soccer but begins to feel tired or suddenly bored, he or she might stop playing. But, if he or she can figure out a way to play anyway, there is a good chance that he or she will feel a little more energized after playing.
3. Guided activity can help a person feel more motivated when symptoms of depression get in the way of motivation. If you wait to become motivated before you do something, you may wait a long time and be unsuccessful in the end. Engaging in activity, even when you don't feel motivated, can actually lead to feeling more motivated. This is called *goal-directed behavior*. Engaging in goal-directed behavior means that you do not wait to feel like doing something before you do it, but you do it because you want to reach a goal or work on feeling better.

Your adolescent's therapist knows that it is hard to engage in activity when feeling depressed, and that it may take a lot of effort for your depressed son or daughter to organize his or her time and engage in activities that may have been fun before but do not now seem interesting. Don't worry; your adolescent's therapist will help him or her figure out the things that get in the way of getting active and will work to help your adolescent break down those roadblocks.

What Will We Be Expected to Do?

There are a couple of things that you and your son or daughter will need to do to make sure treatment is successful.

For your adolescent these include the following:

- Trying to keep all appointments.
- Making an effort to identify things that "trigger" depression.

(continued)

A Parent Guide to Adolescent Depression *(page 3 of 3)*

- Making an effort to work with his or her therapist to set some goals. Making an effort to try some new strategies and activities.
- Being honest with us about what he or she is feeling and what is needed from the therapist.

For parents:

- Trying to keep all appointments—this therapy encourages active involvement of parents and includes time to collaborate with parents to think about new ways to communicate with and support their adolescent.
- Making an effort to recognize and understand your adolescent's depression—how it may affect his or her behavior at home and school.
- Supporting your adolescent in his or her efforts to try new strategies and activities.
- Being honest with us about what you are feeling and what is needed from the therapist.

In summary, the behavioral activation therapist will help your adolescent learn new activities and turn these into new habits that help to improve his or her mood, help him or her engage in the activities that are important, and in turn help to build his or her self-confidence and a sense of purpose.

HANDOUT 7

Getting Active!

Taking Positive Action, even when you are feeling down, can be the first step to feeling better.

MOOD-DIRECTED BEHAVIOR:

Feeling good ⟶ Do something fun, because you feel good ⟶ Feel even better!

MOOD-DIRECTED BEHAVIOR:

Feeling bad ⟶ Do nothing much, because you feel bad ⟶ Feel even worse

GOAL-DIRECTED BEHAVIOR:

Feeling bad ⟶ Do something fun, because you set a goal! ⟶ Feel better

---

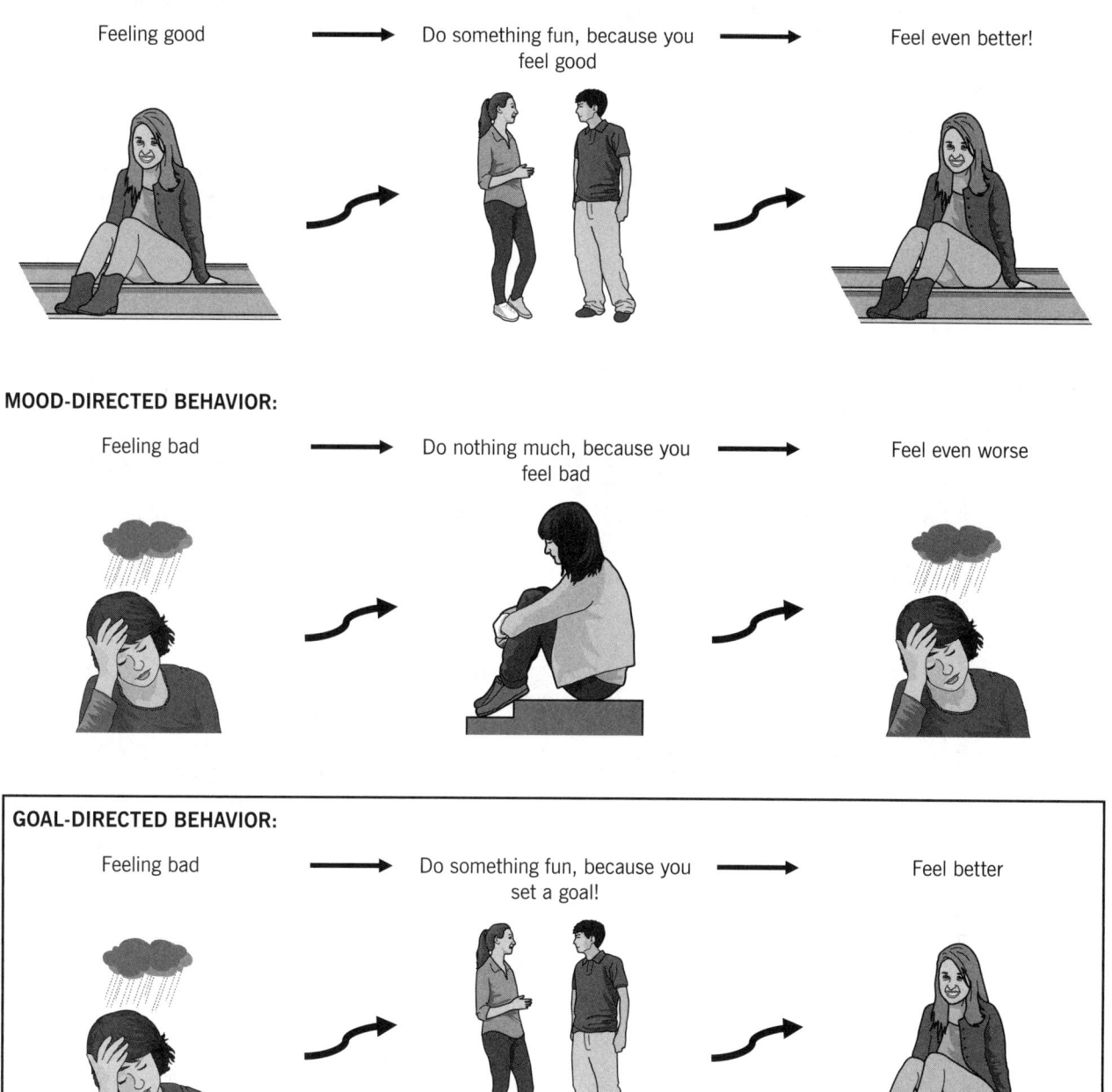

From *Behavioral Activation with Adolescents: A Clinician's Guide* by Elizabeth McCauley, Kelly A. Schloredt, Gretchen R. Gudmundsen, Christopher R. Martell, and Sona Dimidjian. Copyright © 2016 The Guilford Press. Permission to photocopy this handout is granted to purchasers of this book for personal use or use with individual clients (see copyright page for details). Purchasers can download additional copies of this handout (see the box at the end of the table of contents).

HANDOUT 8

Activity–Mood Chart—Example

Example and Practice: Fill in your day so far, including what you were doing, what you were feeling, and the intensity of the feeling.

1	2	3	4	5	6	7	8	9	10
"Not good" (sad, mad, bored)				"Pretty good"					"Great" (happy, engaged)

	Date/Day: Tuesday, June 5	Overall Rating: 6		Date/Day:	Overall Rating:
	Activity	Feeling and Intensity		Activity	Feeling and Intensity
6 AM	Wake up, hit snooze button, shower	Irritated—9	6 AM		
7 AM	Eat breakfast, walk to bus, sat with Allie	A little happy—2	7 AM		
8 AM	Science class/quiz	Anxious—4	8 AM		
9 AM	Language Arts	Relieved—2	9 AM		
10 AM	History	Bored—2	10 AM		
11 AM	Lunch with Jason	Good—6	11 AM		
NOON	Outside after lunch, with Jason and a bunch of his friends	Part good (6), part nervous and lonely (3)	NOON		
1 PM	Math	Bored—5	1 PM		
2 PM	Art	Pretty good—4	2 PM		
3 PM	Bus home, sat alone	Lonely—3	3 PM		
4 PM	Snack, on computer	Okay, a little lonely—3	4 PM		
5 PM	Dad home, nagged	Annoyed—8	5 PM		
6 PM	Dinner, did dishes	Annoyed—6	6 PM		
7 PM	Started homework	Nervous, bored, annoyed—5	7 PM		
8 PM	Homework and on phone a bit	Bored and nervous—4	8 PM		
9 PM	Music, read, played game	Happy—6	9 PM		
10 PM	Parents nagging, got ready for bed	Irritated—3	10 PM		
11 PM	In bed, not falling asleep	Anxious, annoyed—4	11 PM		
12+	Asleep	?	12+		

From *Behavioral Activation with Adolescents: A Clinician's Guide* by Elizabeth McCauley, Kelly A. Schloredt, Gretchen R. Gudmundsen, Christopher R. Martell, and Sona Dimidjian. Copyright © 2016 The Guilford Press. Permission to photocopy this handout is granted to purchasers of this book for personal use or use with individual clients (see copyright page for details). Purchasers can download additional copies of this handout (see the box at the end of the table of contents).

HANDOUT 9

Activity–Mood Chart

Here's what to do:

- Choose 2 days in the week (1 weekday/1 weekend day).
- Keep track of your activities.
- Fill in what you were doing and then . . . .
- Rate how you were feeling (what feeling and how strong):

```
   1    2    3    4    5    6    7    8    9    10
"Not good"      "Pretty good"            "Great"
(sad, mad, bored)                   (happy, engaged)
```

Date/Day:		Overall Rating:
	Activity	Feeling and Intensity
6 AM		
7 AM		
8 AM		
9 AM		
10 AM		
11 AM		
NOON		
1 PM		
2 PM		
3 PM		
4 PM		
5 PM		
6 PM		
7 PM		
8 PM		
9 PM		
10 PM		
11 PM		
12+		

Date/Day:		Overall Rating:
	Activity	Feeling and Intensity
6 AM		
7 AM		
8 AM		
9 AM		
10 AM		
11 AM		
NOON		
1 PM		
2 PM		
3 PM		
4 PM		
5 PM		
6 PM		
7 PM		
8 PM		
9 PM		
10 PM		
11 PM		
12+		

From *Behavioral Activation with Adolescents: A Clinician's Guide* by Elizabeth McCauley, Kelly A. Schloredt, Gretchen R. Gudmundsen, Christopher R. Martell, and Sona Dimidjian. Copyright © 2016 The Guilford Press. Permission to photocopy this handout is granted to purchasers of this book for personal use or use with individual clients (see copyright page for details). Purchasers can download additional copies of this handout (see the box at the end of the table of contents).

HANDOUT 10

Ways to Describe Parenting an Adolescent

Lively - Challenging - **Confusing**

Exciting - Scary - Fun - Hard

Tiring - Unforgettable - **Awesome**

Lonely - **Frustrating** - Bittersweet

Unique - Boring - Sad - **Difficult**

Energizing - **Draining** - Engaging

Never Dull - Thrilling - **Important**

Heart Rending - Wonderful - Painful

Nostalgic - Endearing - **Forever**

Infuriating - **Creative** - Oppressive

Special - Loving - Work - Hopeful

Hopeless - **Impossible** - Admirable

Based on the University of Washington Reconnecting Youth Project.

From *Behavioral Activation with Adolescents: A Clinician's Guide* by Elizabeth McCauley, Kelly A. Schloredt, Gretchen R. Gudmundsen, Christopher R. Martell, and Sona Dimidjian. Copyright © 2016 The Guilford Press. Permission to photocopy this handout is granted to purchasers of this book for personal use or use with individual clients (see copyright page for details). Purchasers can download additional copies of this handout (see the box at the end of the table of contents).

HANDOUT 11

Short- versus Long-Term Consequences

LONG-TERM CONSEQUENCES

	PAYOFF	**PRICE**
SHORT-TERM CONSEQUENCES — PAYOFF	Short-Term Payoff + Long-Term Payoff = **$**	Short-Term Payoff + Long-Term Price = **?** **EVALUATE**
SHORT-TERM CONSEQUENCES — PRICE	Short-Term Price + Long-Term Payoff = **?** **EVALUATE**	Short-Term Price + Long-Term Price = 🚫

From *Behavioral Activation with Adolescents: A Clinician's Guide* by Elizabeth McCauley, Kelly A. Schloredt, Gretchen R. Gudmundsen, Christopher R. Martell, and Sona Dimidjian. Copyright © 2016 The Guilford Press. Permission to photocopy this handout is granted to purchasers of this book for personal use or use with individual clients (see copyright page for details). Purchasers can download additional copies of this handout (see the box at the end of the table of contents).

HANDOUT 12

Pump You Up, Bring You Down

List activities that you can use to **pump yourself up**:

1. _____
2. _____
3. _____
4. _____
5. _____
6. _____
7. _____
8. _____
9. _____
10. _____
11. _____

List activities that **bring you down**:

1. _____
2. _____
3. _____
4. _____
5. _____
6. _____
7. _____
8. _____
9. _____
10. _____
11. _____

From *Behavioral Activation with Adolescents: A Clinician's Guide* by Elizabeth McCauley, Kelly A. Schloredt, Gretchen R. Gudmundsen, Christopher R. Martell, and Sona Dimidjian. Copyright © 2016 The Guilford Press. Permission to photocopy this handout is granted to purchasers of this book for personal use or use with individual clients (see copyright page for details). Purchasers can download additional copies of this handout (see the box at the end of the table of contents).

HANDOUT 13

Activities Menu

Go for a walk	Write a letter to a friend	Draw a picture
Read a good book	Sit and think	Clean the house
Write in a journal	Listen to the birds	Clean the yard
Play with a pet	Go to a movie	Walk by a lake or river
Talk on the phone	Listen to a new radio station	Rent a video
Watch a favorite TV show	Go on a date	Make a new friend
Listen to music	Invite a friend over	Get up extra early
Meditate	Make a silly gift	Sleep extra late
Wear my favorite clothes	Trade back rubs with a friend	Sit beside a waterfall
Clean my room	Be nice to my neighbor	Watch people at the mall
Make something	Go for a hike	Roast marshmallows
Plant something	Help a friend	Sing
Take a hot bath	Try something new	Ride on a ferris wheel
Write a story	Daydream	Talk about religion
Throw a Frisbee	Cook a meal for someone	Finish a project
Play sports	Do someone a favor	Listen to nature
Laugh	Read a newspaper	Dance
Cry	Go for a car ride	Join a group
Play a video game	Wash and wax the car	Think about a world issue
Walk through the mall	Take the bus somewhere	List all of my good points
Do some volunteer work	Go for a walk in the park	Give someone a small gift
Make my favorite snack	Help someone with a project	Go bowling
Take a nap	Pray	Work out
Sit in the sun	Take a dog for a walk	Go for a bike ride
Be with friends	Watch the flowers grow	Find a new band to listen to
Count the stars	Paint your nails	Go see live music
Take a photograph	Decorate your room	Do a handstand
Make a new playlist	Reconnect with an old friend	Try a new food

From *Behavioral Activation with Adolescents: A Clinician's Guide* by Elizabeth McCauley, Kelly A. Schloredt, Gretchen R. Gudmundsen, Christopher R. Martell, and Sona Dimidjian. Copyright © 2016 The Guilford Press. Permission to photocopy this handout is granted to purchasers of this book for personal use or use with individual clients (see copyright page for details). Purchasers can download additional copies of this handout (see the box at the end of the table of contents).

HANDOUT 14

Activities That Help to PUMP You UP!!

What works for YOU?

1. List activities that you can use to pump yourself up.
2. Keep track of what you try and how it works.
3. Don't forget to think about and describe both the short- and long-term consequences and the payoff and the price.
4. Keep track of times when you tried to "make the most of good feelings" and describe how it impacted your mood.

Pump You Up activity	When will you do it?	Did you do it?	How did it impact your mood? What were the short- and long-term consequences, including the payoff and price?
1.			
2.			
3.			
4.			
5.			

Practice making the most of good feelings. Describe what you try, including the situation and what you did to "make the most of it."		How did it impact your mood?
1.		
2.		
3.		

From *Behavioral Activation with Adolescents: A Clinician's Guide* by Elizabeth McCauley, Kelly A. Schloredt, Gretchen R. Gudmundsen, Christopher R. Martell, and Sona Dimidjian. Copyright © 2016 The Guilford Press. Permission to photocopy this handout is granted to purchasers of this book for personal use or use with individual clients (see copyright page for details). Purchasers can download additional copies of this handout (see the box at the end of the table of contents).

HANDOUT 15

Using COPE to Solve Problems

Triggers are situations, feelings, or people that give rise to strong emotions and can "trigger" a response that can get you in trouble or make the problem worse. COPE helps us develop a plan to solve problems, especially when faced with strong emotions.

What are some of your triggers?

_____   _____   _____
_____   _____   _____
_____   _____   _____
_____   _____   _____
_____   _____   _____

Practice: Name a TRIGGER or problem situation: _____

_____

Use COPE to figure out what to do to solve this problem:

C STEP 1: C CALM and CLARIFY

- ✓ STOP before you act.
- ✓ Take deep breaths/count to 10.
- ✓ Clarify what is TRIGGERING your feelings and what is the real problem!

O STEP 2: O Figure out your OPTIONS

- ✓ What can you do to feel better *and* keep moving toward your goal?

P STEP 3: P PERFORM

- ✓ Pick a solution and try it out!

E STEP 4: E EVALUATE

- ✓ How did it work?
- ✓ If helpful, keep it up; if not, test out a different option.

From *Behavioral Activation with Adolescents: A Clinician's Guide* by Elizabeth McCauley, Kelly A. Schloredt, Gretchen R. Gudmundsen, Christopher R. Martell, and Sona Dimidjian. Copyright © 2016 The Guilford Press. Permission to photocopy this handout is granted to purchasers of this book for personal use or use with individual clients (see copyright page for details). Purchasers can download additional copies of this handout (see the box at the end of the table of contents).

HANDOUT 16

Using COPE

Describe a Trigger Situation . . . _____

_____
_____
_____
_____
_____
_____
_____

Then use COPE . . .

C STEP 1: CALM and CLARIFY

- ✓ STOP before you act.
- ✓ Take deep breaths/count to 10.
- ✓ Clarify what is TRIGGERING your feelings and what is the real problem!
- ✓ Describe the real problem (same as trigger or something else): ____

O STEP 2: Figure out your OPTIONS

What can you do to feel better *and* also keep moving toward your goal?

_____   _____
_____   _____
_____   _____
_____   _____
_____   _____

P STEP 3: PERFORM

- ✓ Pick a solution.
- ✓ Troubleshoot obstacles.
- ✓ Try it out!

E STEP 4: EVALUATE

- ✓ How did it work? _____

_____.

- ✓ If helpful keep it up, if not, test out a different option.

New option to try: _____

_____.

From *Behavioral Activation with Adolescents: A Clinician's Guide* by Elizabeth McCauley, Kelly A. Schloredt, Gretchen R. Gudmundsen, Christopher R. Martell, and Sona Dimidjian. Copyright © 2016 The Guilford Press. Permission to photocopy this handout is granted to purchasers of this book for personal use or use with individual clients (see copyright page for details). Purchasers can download additional copies of this handout (see the box at the end of the table of contents).

HANDOUT 17

How to Communicate with Support

The Active Listener . . .

- ✓ Gives the speaker the floor.
- ✓ Looks interested . . .
    - Good eye contact
    - Stops to listen
    - Indicates understanding . . . "Uh-huh"
- ✓ Asks CLARIFYING QUESTIONS . . .
    - Do you mean . . . ?
    - Can you tell me about . . . ?
- ✓ Reflects FEELINGS . . .
    - It sounds as though you feel . . .
    - Wow! It sounds like that makes you . . .
    - It looks to me like you are . . .
- ✓ Paraphrases . . .
    - "I hear you saying . . ."
    - "So, in other words . . ."
    - "It seems. . . . Is that right?"

The Active Listener Does NOT . . .

Interrupt
Discount what's being said
Argue
Give unwanted advice
Criticize
Engage in another activity
Make judgments
Space out
Talk about him- or herself

Note. Based on Eggert, Nicholas, and Owens (1995).

From *Behavioral Activation with Adolescents: A Clinician's Guide* by Elizabeth McCauley, Kelly A. Schloredt, Gretchen R. Gudmundsen, Christopher R. Martell, and Sona Dimidjian. Copyright © 2016 The Guilford Press. Permission to photocopy this handout is granted to purchasers of this book for personal use or use with individual clients (see copyright page for details). Purchasers can download additional copies of this handout (see the box at the end of the table of contents).

HANDOUT 18

Practicing How to Communicate with Support

Remember, a parent can show support by:
- ✓ Giving the speaker the floor
- ✓ Showing interest
- ✓ Asking clarifying questions
- ✓ Reflecting feelings
- ✓ Paraphrasing to show that he or she is listening

Practice: What can you say in the following situations to show support?

The adolescent is looking through a pile of books, looking overwhelmed. Tells the parent he or she has a major assignment due in just a few days. _____

_____

_____

_____

Parent is busy doing the dishes; adolescent comes in and with a loud sigh throws his or her books on table. _____

_____

_____

_____

Adolescent declares that he or she is going to drop math because the "teacher just doesn't like me, so I'll never pass." _____

_____

_____

_____

Adolescent stuck at home after not being invited to a friend's party. _____

_____

_____

_____

Adolescent gets stopped by the police for speeding. _____

_____

_____

_____

From *Behavioral Activation with Adolescents: A Clinician's Guide* by Elizabeth McCauley, Kelly A. Schloredt, Gretchen R. Gudmundsen, Christopher R. Martell, and Sona Dimidjian. Copyright © 2016 The Guilford Press. Permission to photocopy this handout is granted to purchasers of this book for personal use or use with individual clients (see copyright page for details). Purchasers can download additional copies of this handout (see the box at the end of the table of contents).

HANDOUT 19

Communicating with Support: What Can You Do to Help an Interaction Go Well?

Outline a situation with your adolescent in which communication was difficult and did not go well . . .	Outline a situation with your adolescent in which communication was positive and went really well . . .
1. What was the situation? _____ _____ _____ 2. How did you show support? _____ _____ _____ 3. How did your adolescent respond? _____ _____ _____	1. What was the situation? _____ _____ _____ 2. How did you show support? _____ _____ _____ 3. How did your adolescent respond? _____ _____ _____

Comparing the two situations and your adolescent's response, what did you learn? _____
_____
_____
_____

What can you commit to work on with regard to improving communication with your adolescent? _____
_____
_____
_____

From *Behavioral Activation with Adolescents: A Clinician's Guide* by Elizabeth McCauley, Kelly A. Schloredt, Gretchen R. Gudmundsen, Christopher R. Martell, and Sona Dimidjian. Copyright © 2016 The Guilford Press. Permission to photocopy this handout is granted to purchasers of this book for personal use or use with individual clients (see copyright page for details). Purchasers can download additional copies of this handout (see the box at the end of the table of contents).

HANDOUT 20

Setting SMART Goals

> **Effective goals are SMART goals:**
> - ✓ Specific—Clear and specifically stated, describing what you will do.
> - ✓ Measurable—Include an easy way to identify whether or not it was accomplished.
> - ✓ Appealing—Desirable, something you value, a healthy choice.
> - ✓ Realistic—Achievable, controllable, within reach but not too easy.
> - ✓ Time-bound—Do not go on endlessly, but have a clear start and finish.

Once you have identified your SMART goal . . .

Take the mini-steps to success by breaking it down into something doable.

Example: If you are having a hard time getting your homework done—setting the goal of achieving a 4.0 GPA by the end of term would involve too big a step to start with. It would not be SMART.

But . . .

Making a plan to get your math homework completed and turned in for the next 3 days would be SMART and includes the mini-steps to start you in the right direction.

Practice by identifying a SMART goal you would like to work on over the next few weeks: _____
_____
_____
_____

Does it meet your SMART requirements?

Note. Based on Doran (1981).

From *Behavioral Activation with Adolescents: A Clinician's Guide* by Elizabeth McCauley, Kelly A. Schloredt, Gretchen R. Gudmundsen, Christopher R. Martell, and Sona Dimidjian. Copyright © 2016 The Guilford Press. Permission to photocopy this handout is granted to purchasers of this book for personal use or use with individual clients (see copyright page for details). Purchasers can download additional copies of this handout (see the box at the end of the table of contents).

HANDOUT 21

How SMART Is This Goal?

> Remember, a SMART goal is:
> - ✓ Specific—Clear and specifically stated, describing what you will do.
> - ✓ Measurable—Includes an easy way to identify whether or not it was accomplished.
> - ✓ Appealing—Desirable, something you value, a healthy choice.
> - ✓ Realistic—Achievable, controllable, within reach but not *too* easy.
> - ✓ Time-bound—Does not go on endlessly, but has a clear start and finish.

How SMART Is This Goal?	Specific	Measurable	Appealing	Realistic	Time-Bound
To go to the mall with my sister once this week?					
To get along with my parents?					
To ask my brother to help me practice soccer/baseball before my game on Saturday?					
To become a famous movie star/rock star/professional sports player?					
To not have to talk with my parents about anything ever again?					
To get a "B" or above on my math quiz on Friday?					
To quit school?					

Note. Based on Doran (1981).

From *Behavioral Activation with Adolescents: A Clinician's Guide* by Elizabeth McCauley, Kelly A. Schloredt, Gretchen R. Gudmundsen, Christopher R. Martell, and Sona Dimidjian. Copyright © 2016 The Guilford Press. Permission to photocopy this handout is granted to purchasers of this book for personal use or use with individual clients (see copyright page for details). Purchasers can download additional copies of this handout (see the box at the end of the table of contents).

HANDOUT 22

Identifying a SMART Goal

What is important to you? Identify which factors would be the focus of a SMART goal that would help you feel better or improve your situation? What would be the focus of your first goal?

What might be important in each of these areas that could help you identify a goal for the next week that can give you a boost?

- In school _____
- With friends _____
- With family _____
- During activities (sports, music, etc.) _____
- Other _____

Which area do you want to focus on for your first goal? _____
_____

From *Behavioral Activation with Adolescents: A Clinician's Guide* by Elizabeth McCauley, Kelly A. Schloredt, Gretchen R. Gudmundsen, Christopher R. Martell, and Sona Dimidjian. Copyright © 2016 The Guilford Press. Permission to photocopy this handout is granted to purchasers of this book for personal use or use with individual clients (see copyright page for details). Purchasers can download additional copies of this handout (see the box at the end of the table of contents).

HANDOUT 23

Goal Setting

Remember a SMART goal is:

- ✓ **Specific**—Clear and specifically stated, describing what you will do.
- ✓ **Measurable**—Includes an easy way to identify whether or not it was accomplished.
- ✓ **Appealing**—Desirable, something you value, a healthy choice.
- ✓ **Realistic**—Achievable, controllable, within reach but not too easy.
- ✓ **Time-bound**—Does not go on endlessly, but has a clear start and finish.

My Goal is: _____

Who can help me? _____

Mini-Step 1: _____
When will I do this? _____
What happened? _____

Mini-Step 2: _____
When will I do this? _____
What happened? _____

Mini-Step 3: _____
When will I do this? _____
What happened? _____

Mini-Step 4: _____
When will I do this? _____
What happened? _____

Note. Based on Doran (1981).

From *Behavioral Activation with Adolescents: A Clinician's Guide* by Elizabeth McCauley, Kelly A. Schloredt, Gretchen R. Gudmundsen, Christopher R. Martell, and Sona Dimidjian. Copyright © 2016 The Guilford Press. Permission to photocopy this handout is granted to purchasers of this book for personal use or use with individual clients (see copyright page for details). Purchasers can download additional copies of this handout (see the box at the end of the table of contents).

HANDOUT 24

Ways to Support My Adolescent

- Give your adolescent space when he or she asks for it.
- Listen—Did you use active listening?
- Ask questions to find out more about the situation.
- Show your concern and that you are trying to understand his or her perspective.
- Acknowledge all positive or healthy choices you see.
- Praise steps in the right direction (even little steps).
- Express confidence in your adolescent.
- Remind the adolescent of his or her good qualities, strengths, and attributes you value.
- Encourage your adolescent to do his or her best.
- Say please and thank you!
- Model healthy problem solving.
- Take time to compliment your child. Use specific compliments (e.g., "I especially like that you took some of your lunch break to check in with your Algebra teacher").
- Be willing to drive your child to activities, friends' houses, or other healthy "pump you up" activities.

Other Ideas:

1. _____
2. _____
3. _____

From *Behavioral Activation with Adolescents: A Clinician's Guide* by Elizabeth McCauley, Kelly A. Schloredt, Gretchen R. Gudmundsen, Christopher R. Martell, and Sona Dimidjian. Copyright © 2016 The Guilford Press. Permission to photocopy this handout is granted to purchasers of this book for personal use or use with individual clients (see copyright page for details). Purchasers can download additional copies of this handout (see the box at the end of the table of contents).

HANDOUT 25

Monitoring Support

Select two support goals for the next week. Please keep track of how it goes, and at the end of the week please rate your progress. Remember, monitoring is one of the first steps toward reaching a goal.

Goal 1. I will support my teen by _____

_____

_____.

Right before our next session, please consider your support goal and rate how often you were able to show support in the last week:

    5 = Used every opportunity to be supportive
    4 = Took advantage of many opportunities
    3 = Used about half of the support opportunities
    2 = Occasionally found opportunities to be supportive
    1 = Did not find opportunities to be supportive

Goal 2. I will support my teen by _____

_____

_____.

Right before our next session, please consider your support goal and rate how often you were able to show support in the last week:

    5 = Used every opportunity to be supportive
    4 = Took advantage of many opportunities
    3 = Used about half of the support opportunities
    2 = Occasionally found opportunities to be supportive
    1 = Did not find opportunities to be supportive

From *Behavioral Activation with Adolescents: A Clinician's Guide* by Elizabeth McCauley, Kelly A. Schloredt, Gretchen R. Gudmundsen, Christopher R. Martell, and Sona Dimidjian. Copyright © 2016 The Guilford Press. Permission to photocopy this handout is granted to purchasers of this book for personal use or use with individual clients (see copyright page for details). Purchasers can download additional copies of this handout (see the box at the end of the table of contents).

HANDOUT 26

Barriers: Internal versus External

Internal Barriers: Things that are "inside of us," such as thoughts and feelings that prevent or stop us from completing our goals.

Examples:

☐ Just don't feel like it/unmotivated

☐ Difficulty communicating and/or getting what I need

☐ Let myself get distracted—video games, Facebook, watching movies or TV

☐ Feel overwhelmed

☐ _____

☐ _____

I will get around this by: _____

_____

_____

External Barriers: Things that are "outside of us," that prevent us from achieving our goals, such as not having enough time, money, or the necessary tools.

Examples:

☐ Not having the necessary "tools" (e.g., don't have assignment, can't get book)

☐ Need help from others to carry out plan (e.g., ride from father, quiet time at home, tutor/homework help)

☐ Other people changing plans or not following through

☐ Need money

☐ _____

☐ _____

I will get around this by: _____

_____

_____

From *Behavioral Activation with Adolescents: A Clinician's Guide* by Elizabeth McCauley, Kelly A. Schloredt, Gretchen R. Gudmundsen, Christopher R. Martell, and Sona Dimidjian. Copyright © 2016 The Guilford Press. Permission to photocopy this handout is granted to purchasers of this book for personal use or use with individual clients (see copyright page for details). Purchasers can download additional copies of this handout (see the box at the end of the table of contents).

HANDOUT 27

Goals and Barriers

Remember a SMART goal is:

- ✓ **Specific**—Clear and specifically stated, describing what you will do.
- ✓ **Measurable**—Includes an easy way to identify whether or not it was accomplished.
- ✓ **Appealing**—Desirable, something you value, a healthy choice.
- ✓ **Realistic**—Achievable, controllable, within reach but not too easy.
- ✓ **Time-bound**—Does not go on endlessly, but has a clear start and finish.

My Goal is: _____

Who can help me? _____

Mini-Step 1: _____
When will I do this? _____
Barriers to Overcome? _____
What happened? _____

Mini-Step 2: _____
When will I do this? _____
Barriers to Overcome? _____
What happened? _____

Mini-Step 3: _____
When will I do this? _____
Barriers to Overcome? _____
What happened? _____

Mini-Step 4: _____
When will I do this? _____
Barriers to Overcome? _____
What happened? _____

Note. Based on Doran (1981).

From *Behavioral Activation with Adolescents: A Clinician's Guide* by Elizabeth McCauley, Kelly A. Schloredt, Gretchen R. Gudmundsen, Christopher R. Martell, and Sona Dimidjian. Copyright © 2016 The Guilford Press. Permission to photocopy this handout is granted to purchasers of this book for personal use or use with individual clients (see copyright page for details). Purchasers can download additional copies of this handout (see the box at the end of the table of contents).

HANDOUT 28

Support Ideas

✓ Give space.

✓ Listen.

✓ Find out more about the situation.

✓ Show your concern.

✓ Acknowledge the child's effort.

✓ Praise steps in the right direction.

✓ Express confidence.

✓ Point out good qualities, strengths, and attributes you value.

✓ Be encouraging.

✓ Say please and thank you.

✓ Be flexible.

✓ Offer to help when you can (e.g., projects, transportation, having friends over).

Other Ideas:

1. _____
2. _____
3. _____

From *Behavioral Activation with Adolescents: A Clinician's Guide* by Elizabeth McCauley, Kelly A. Schloredt, Gretchen R. Gudmundsen, Christopher R. Martell, and Sona Dimidjian. Copyright © 2016 The Guilford Press. Permission to photocopy this handout is granted to purchasers of this book for personal use or use with individual clients (see copyright page for details). Purchasers can download additional copies of this handout (see the box at the end of the table of contents).

HANDOUT 29

Support Experiment

I will support my adolescent by: _____

_____

_____

Keep track of how it goes . . .

Tracking Parent Support							
Day:	1	2	3	4	5	6	7
Used every opportunity to be supportive	5	5	5	5	5	5	5
Took advantage of many opportunities	4	4	4	4	4	4	4
Used about half of the support opportunities	3	3	3	3	3	3	3
Occasionally found opportunities to be supportive	2	2	2	2	2	2	2
Did not find opportunities to be supportive	1	1	1	1	1	1	1

From *Behavioral Activation with Adolescents: A Clinician's Guide* by Elizabeth McCauley, Kelly A. Schloredt, Gretchen R. Gudmundsen, Christopher R. Martell, and Sona Dimidjian. Copyright © 2016 The Guilford Press. Permission to photocopy this handout is granted to purchasers of this book for personal use or use with individual clients (see copyright page for details). Purchasers can download additional copies of this handout (see the box at the end of the table of contents).

HANDOUT 30

What Does Avoidance Look Like?

Avoidance comes in all sizes and shapes . . .

- **Procrastinating**—Putting off necessary or boring tasks, waiting until the last minute to start your paper.

- **Brooding**—Thinking over and over about a problem without coming to any solution.

- **Bursting**—Blowing up at people or things, trying to get people off your back by yelling or throwing a tantrum.

- **Hibernating**—Shutting down from everything, staying in bed all day, withdrawing from friends.

What does Avoidance look like for you? _____

_____

_____

_____

_____

Remember:

- **Avoidance can have a short PAYOFF, but a long-term PRICE.**
- **Avoidance can be a negative TRAP.**

From *Behavioral Activation with Adolescents: A Clinician's Guide* by Elizabeth McCauley, Kelly A. Schloredt, Gretchen R. Gudmundsen, Christopher R. Martell, and Sona Dimidjian. Copyright © 2016 The Guilford Press. Permission to photocopy this handout is granted to purchasers of this book for personal use or use with individual clients (see copyright page for details). Purchasers can download additional copies of this handout (see the box at the end of the table of contents).

HANDOUT 31

Using TRAP-TRAC to Conquer Avoidance and Overcome the Downward Spiral

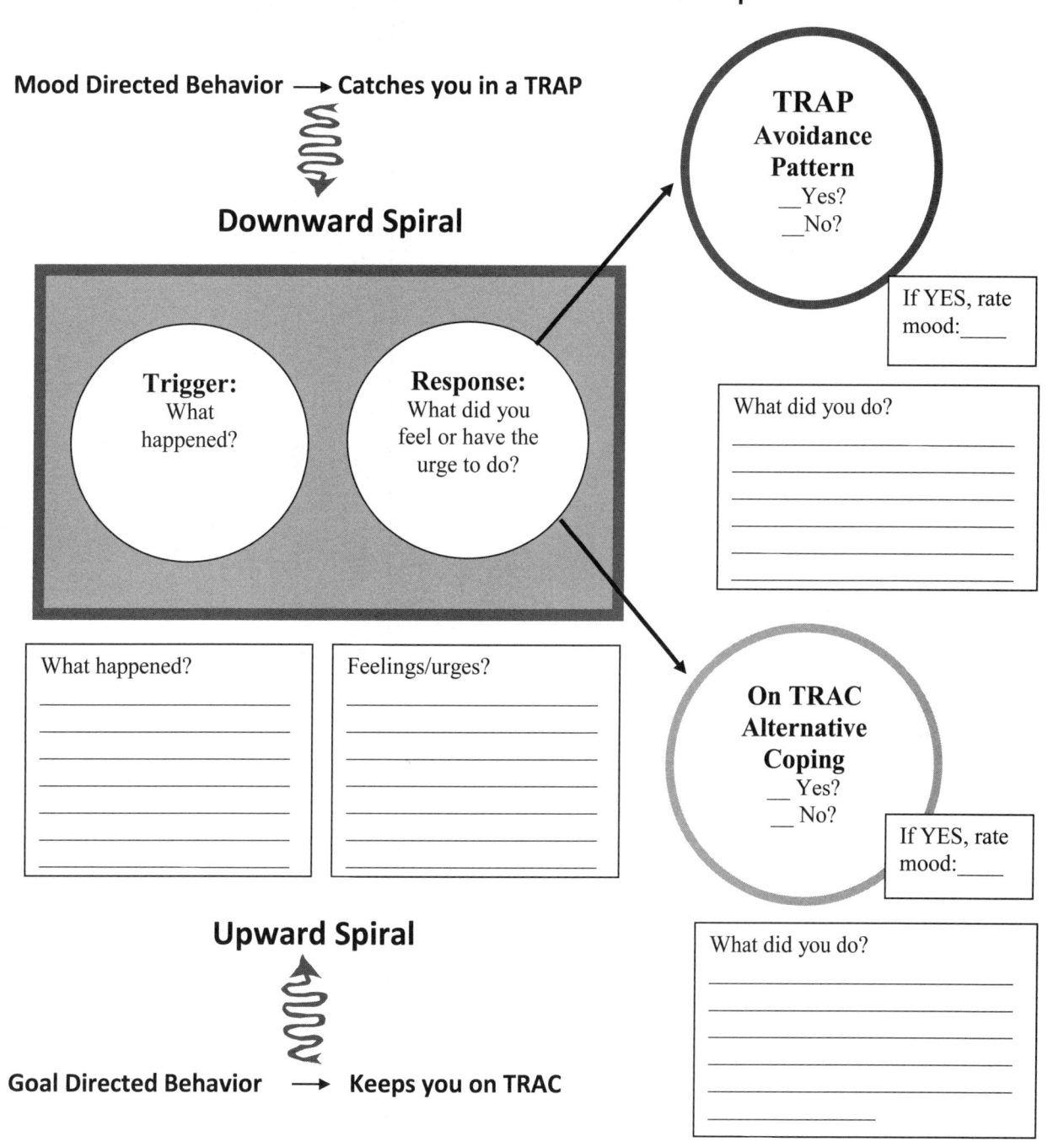

Mood Directed Behavior → Catches you in a TRAP

Downward Spiral

Trigger: What happened?

Response: What did you feel or have the urge to do?

TRAP Avoidance Pattern
__Yes?
__No?

If YES, rate mood:____

What did you do?
_____
_____
_____
_____
_____

What happened?
_____
_____
_____
_____
_____

Feelings/urges?
_____
_____
_____
_____
_____

On TRAC Alternative Coping
__Yes?
__No?

If YES, rate mood:____

What did you do?
_____
_____
_____
_____
_____
_____

Upward Spiral

Goal Directed Behavior → Keeps you on TRAC

From *Behavioral Activation with Adolescents: A Clinician's Guide* by Elizabeth McCauley, Kelly A. Schloredt, Gretchen R. Gudmundsen, Christopher R. Martell, and Sona Dimidjian. Copyright © 2016 The Guilford Press. Permission to photocopy this handout is granted to purchasers of this book for personal use or use with individual clients (see copyright page for details). Purchasers can download additional copies of this handout (see the box at the end of the table of contents).

HANDOUT 32

Taking Stock

Where have you been with your mood?

| At the Start | Midtreatment | Now | End |

Where do things stand now?

- In school _____
- With friends _____
- With family _____
- During activities (sports, music, etc.) _____
- What do you want to focus on? _____

From *Behavioral Activation with Adolescents: A Clinician's Guide* by Elizabeth McCauley, Kelly A. Schloredt, Gretchen R. Gudmundsen, Christopher R. Martell, and Sona Dimidjian. Copyright © 2016 The Guilford Press. Permission to photocopy this handout is granted to purchasers of this book for personal use or use with individual clients (see copyright page for details). Purchasers can download additional copies of this handout (see the box at the end of the table of contents).

HANDOUT 33

Developing an Action Plan

My Goal for the next week is: _____

Who can help me? _____

What can I use to help me move toward my goal:
- What **"Pump You Up"** activities can help me? _____
- What are my **Triggers** for using **COPE**? _____
- How can I be sure to make the most of a **GOOD Moment**? _____
- What **Barriers** will pop up? How will I overcome them? _____
- What does **AVOIDANCE** look like for me?

  Procrastinating ____ Brooding ____ Bursting ____ Hibernating ____ Other Ways of Avoiding ____

- What **Alternative Coping** strategies will I use to stay **GOAL**-directed, not mood-directed, and overcome avoidance? _____

Mini-Steps toward my Goal:

Mini-Step 1: _____
When will I do this? _____
Barriers to Overcome? _____
What happened? _____

Mini-Step 2: _____
When will I do this? _____
Barriers to Overcome? _____
What happened? _____

Mini-Step 3: _____
When will I do this? _____
Barriers to Overcome? _____
What happened? _____

Mini-Step 4: _____
When will I do this? _____
Barriers to Overcome? _____
What happened? _____

From *Behavioral Activation with Adolescents: A Clinician's Guide* by Elizabeth McCauley, Kelly A. Schloredt, Gretchen R. Gudmundsen, Christopher R. Martell, and Sona Dimidjian. Copyright © 2016 The Guilford Press. Permission to photocopy this handout is granted to purchasers of this book for personal use or use with individual clients (see copyright page for details). Purchasers can download additional copies of this handout (see the box at the end of the table of contents).

HANDOUT 34

Action Plan

Keep track of what you are doing and how you are feeling:

- Schedule when to work on mini-steps to reach your GOALS.
- Plan "Pump You Up" activities.
- Evaluate the PAYOFF versus PRICE, short term and long term.
- Use "COPE" when faced with problems.
- Goal-directed, not mood-directed behavior.
- Make the most of good moments.
- Anticipate barriers and work around them.
- Be aware of Avoidance.
- Use Alternative Coping.

	Monday	Tuesday	Wednesday	Thursday	Friday	Saturday	Sunday
6–8 AM							
8–10 AM							
10–12 PM							
12–2 PM							
2–4 PM							
4–6 PM							
6–8 PM							
8–10 PM							
10–12 PM							
12–6 AM							

From *Behavioral Activation with Adolescents: A Clinician's Guide* by Elizabeth McCauley, Kelly A. Schloredt, Gretchen R. Gudmundsen, Christopher R. Martell, and Sona Dimidjian. Copyright © 2016 The Guilford Press. Permission to photocopy this handout is granted to purchasers of this book for personal use or use with individual clients (see copyright page for details). Purchasers can download additional copies of this handout (see the box at the end of the table of contents).

HANDOUT 35

Doing What Works

Triggers (vulnerable situations)

Disappointments _____

Big Changes _____

Frustrations _____

Other _____

_____

_____

Signs of Slipping (how you feel, what you do)

Feelings _____

Body Signs _____

Avoidant Behaviors _____

Risky Behaviors _____

Other _____

_____

_____

What to do if you SLIP:

☐ Mini-steps to reach your GOALS

☐ Making the most of GOOD moments

☐ Evaluate the PAYOFF versus PRICE, short term and long term

☐ Use "COPE" when faced with problems

☐ Plan and do "PUMP You UP" activities

☐ Recognizing TRAPs and using Alternative Coping or skills

Who will I ask for support and/or help?

_____   _____

_____   _____

From *Behavioral Activation with Adolescents: A Clinician's Guide* by Elizabeth McCauley, Kelly A. Schloredt, Gretchen R. Gudmundsen, Christopher R. Martell, and Sona Dimidjian. Copyright © 2016 The Guilford Press. Permission to photocopy this handout is granted to purchasers of this book for personal use or use with individual clients (see copyright page for details). Purchasers can download additional copies of this handout (see the box at the end of the table of contents).

References

Aarons, G., & Chaffin, M. (2013, April). Scaling-up evidence-based practices in child welfare services systems: Child welfare system involvement may serve as a gateway for identification of, and services for, mental health problems of youth and parents. *CYF News*, n.p.

Achenbach, T. M. (2009). *The Achenbach System of Empirically Based Assessment (ASEBA): Development, findings, theory, and applications.* Burlington: University of Vermont Research Center for Children, Youth and Families.

Akiskal, H. S. (2007). Toward a definition of generalized anxiety disorder as an anxious temperament type. *Acta Psychiatrica Scandinavica, 98*(Suppl. 393), 66–73.

American Psychiatric Association. (2013). *Diagnostic and statistical manual of mental disorders* (5th ed.). Arlington, VA: Author.

Angold, A., Costello, E. J., & Erkanli, A. (1999). Comorbidity. *Journal of Child Psychiatry and Psychology, 40*, 57–87.

Angold, A., Costello, E. J., Messer, S. C., Pickles, A., Winder, F., & Silver, D. (1995). Development of a short questionnaire for use in epidemiological studies of depression in children and adolescents. *International Journal of Methods in Psychiatric Research, 5*, 237–249.

Barkley, R. A. (2005). *Attention-deficit/hyperactivity disorder: A handbook for diagnosis and treatment* (3rd ed.). New York: Guilford Press.

Baum, W. (2005). *Understanding behaviorism: Behavior, culture, and evolution* (2nd ed.). Malden, MA: Blackwell.

Beck, A. T., Rush, A. J., Shaw, B. F., & Emery, G. (1979). *Cognitive therapy of depression.* New York: Guilford Press.

Becker, K. D., Lee, B. L., Daleiden, E. L., Lindsey, M., Brandt, N. E., & Chorpita, B. F. (2015). The common elements of engagement in children's mental health services: Which elements for which outcomes? *Journal of Clinical Child and Adolescent Psychology, 44*(1), 30–43.

Bickman, L., Kelley, S. D., Breda, C., de Andrade, A. R., & Riemer, M. (2011). Effects of routine feedback to clinicians on mental health outcomes of youths: Results of a randomized trial. *Psychiatric Services, 62*(12), 1423–1429.

Birmaher, B., Ryan, N. D., Williamson, D. E., Brent, D. A., & Kaufman, J. (1996). Childhood and adolescent depression: A review of the past 10 years: Part I. *Journal of the American Academy of Child and Adolescent Psychiatry, 35*(11), 1427–1439.

Brent, D. A., & Birmaher, B. (2004). British warnings on SSRIs questioned. *Journal of the American Academy of Child and Adolescent Psychiatry, 43*(4), 379–380.

Bridge, J. A., Barbe, R. P., Birmaher, B., Kolko, D. J., & Brent, D. A. (2005). Emergent suicidality in a clinical psychotherapy trial for adolescent depression. *American Journal of Psychiatry, 162*(11), 2173–2175.

Burke, J. D., Loeber, R., Lahey, B. B., & Rathouz, P. J. (2005). Developmental transitions among affective and behavioral disorders in adolescent boys. *Journal of Child Psychology and Psychiatry, 46*, 1200–1210.

Burwell, R. A., & Shirk, S. R. (2007). Subtypes of rumination in adolescence: Association between brooding, reflection, depressive symptoms, and coping. *Journal of Clinical Child and Adolescent Psychology, 36*, 56–65.

Busch, A. M., Whited, M. C., Appelhans, B. M., Schneider, K. L., Waring, M. E., DeBiasse, M. A., et al. (2013). Reliable change in depression during behavioral weight loss treatment among women with major depression. *Obesity, 21*(3), E211–E218.

Campbell, D. T., & Fiske, D. W. (1959). Convergent and discriminant validation by the multitrait–multimethod matrix. *Psychological Bulletin, 56*(2), 81–105.

Carlier, I. V. E., Meuldijk, D., Van Vliet, I. M., Van Fenema, E., Van der Wee, N. J. A., & Zitman, F. G. (2012). ROM and feedback on physical or mental health status: Evidence and theory. *Journal of Evaluation in Clinical Practice, 18*, 104–110.

Carskadon, M. A. (Ed.). (2002). *Adolescent sleep patterns: Biological, social and psychological influences*. New York: Cambridge University Press.

Casey, B. J., Duhoux, S., & Cohen, M. M. (2010). Adolescence: What do transmission, transition, and translation have to do with it? *Neuron, 67*(5), 749–760.

Chen, J., Liu, X., Rapee, R. M., & Pillay, P. (2013). Behavioural activation: A pilot trial of transdiagnostic treatment for excessive worry. *Behaviour Research and Therapy, 51*(9), 533–539.

Chorpita, B. F., & Daleiden, E. L. (2009). Mapping evidence-based treatments for children and adolescents: Application of the distillation and matching model to 615 treatments from 322 randomized trials. *Journal of Consulting and Clinical Psychology, 77*(3), 566–579.

Chorpita, B. F., Daleiden, E. L., & Weisz, J. R. (2005). Modularity in the design and application of therapeutic interventions. *Applied and Preventive Psychology, 11*(3), 141–156.

Chu, B. C., Colognori, D., Weissman, A. S., & Bannon, K. (2009). An initial description and pilot of group behavioral activation therapy for anxious and depressed youth. *Cognitive and Behavioral Practice, 16*(4), 408–419.

Clarke, G., DeBar, L., Ludman, E., Asarnow, J., & Jaycox, L. (2002). *STEADY Project intervention manual: Collaborative care, cognitive-behavioral program for depressed youth in a primary care setting*. Retrieved from *www.in.gov/idoc/files/steady_project_intervention1.pdf*.

Clarke, G., Hops, H., Lewinsohn, P. M., Andrews, J., Seeley, J. R., & Williams, J. (1992). Cognitive-behavioral group treatment of adolescent depression: Prediction of outcome. *Behavior Therapy, 23*(3), 341–354.

Cohen, J. A., Mannarino, A. P., & Deblinger, E. (2006). *Treating trauma and traumatic grief in children and adolescents*. New York: Guilford Press.

Copeland, W. E., Shanahan, L., Costello, E. J., & Angold, A. (2009). Childhood and adolescent psychiatric disorders as predictors of young adult disorders. *Archives of General Psychiatry, 66*(7), 764–772.

Costello, E. J., Egger, H., & Angold, A. (2005). 10-year research update review: The epidemiology of child and adolescent psychiatric disorders: I. Methods and public health burden. *Journal of the American Academy of Child and Adolescent Psychiatry, 44*(10), 972–986.

Costello, E. J., Foley, D., & Angold, A. (2006). 10-year research update review: The epidemiology of child and adolescent psychiatric disorders: II. Developmental epidemiology. *Journal of the American Academy of Child Psychiatry, 45*(1), 8–25.

Crone, E. A., Wendelken, C., Donohue, S., van Leijenhorst, L., & Bunge, S. A. (2006). Neurocognitive development of the ability to manipulate information in working memory. *Proceedings of the National Academy of Sciences, 103*(24), 9315–9320.

Curry, J., Silva, S., Rohde, P., Ginsburg, G., Kratochvil, C., Simons, A., et al. (2011). Recovery and recurrence following treatment for adolescent major depression. *Archives of General Psychiatry, 68*(3), 263–269.

Davey, C. G., Yücel, M., & Allen, N. B. (2008). The emergence of depression in adolescence: Development of the prefrontal cortex and the representation of reward. *Neuroscience and Biobehavioral Reviews, 32*(1), 1–19.

David-Ferdon, C., & Kaslow, N. J. (2008). Evidence-based psychosocial treatments for child and adolescent depression. *Journal of Clinical Child and Adolescent Psychology, 37*(1), 62–104.

DeRubeis, R. J., Hollon, S. D., Amsterdam, J. D., Shelton, R. C., Young, P. R., Salomon, R. M., et al. (2005). Cognitive therapy vs medications in the treatment of moderate to severe depression. *Archives of General Psychiatry, 62*, 409–416.

DeRubeis, R. J., Siegle, G. J., & Hollon, S. D. (2008). Cognitive therapy versus medication for depression: Treatment outcomes and neural mechanisms. *Nature Reviews Neuroscience, 9*(10), 788–796.

Diamond, G., & Josephson, A. (2005). Family-based treatment research: A 10-year update. *Journal of the American Academy of Child and Adolescent Psychiatry, 44*(9), 872–887.

Diamond, G. S., Wintersteen, M. B., Brown, G. K., Diamond, G. M., Gallop, R., Shelef, K., et al. (2010). Attachment-based family therapy for adolescents with suicidal ideation: A randomized controlled trial. *Journal of the American Academy of Child and Adolescent Psychiatry, 49*(2), 122–131.

Dimidjian, S., Hollon, S. D., Dobson, K. S., Schmaling, K. B., Kohlenberg, R. J., Addis, M. E., et al. (2006). Randomized trial of behavioral activation, cognitive therapy, and antidepressant medication in the acute treatment of adults with major depression. *Journal of Consulting and Clinical Psychology, 74*(4), 658–670.

Doran, G. T. (1981). There's a SMART way to write management's goals and objectives. *Management Review, 70*(11), 35–36.

Dowell, K. A., & Ogles, B. M. (2010). The effects of parent participation on child psychotherapy outcome: A meta-analytic review. *Journal of Clinical Child and Adolescent Psychology, 39*(2), 151–162.

Dunn, V., & Goodyer, I. M. (2006). Longitudinal investigation into childhood- and adolescence-onset depression: Psychiatric outcome in early adulthood. *British Journal of Psychiatry, 188*(3), 216–222.

Edelbrock, C., Costello, A. J., Dulcan, M. K., Conover, N. C., & Kalas, R. (1986). Parent–child agreement on child psychiatric symptoms assessed via structured interview. *Journal of Child Psychology and Psychiatry, 27*, 181–190.

Eells, T. D. (2007). History and current status of psychotherapy case formulation. In T. D. Eells (Ed.), *Handbook of psychotherapy case formulation* (2nd ed., pp. 3–32). New York: Guilford Press.

Eggert, L. L., Nicholas, L. J., & Owens, L. M. (1995). Reconnecting youth: A peer group approach to building life skills. Bloomington, IN: National Educational Service.

Eltz, M. J., Shirk, S. R., & Sarlin, N. (1995). Alliance formation and treatment outcome among maltreated adolescents. *Child Abuse and Neglect, 19*(4), 419–431.

Fergusson, D. M., & Woodward, L. J. (2002). Mental health, educational, and social role outcomes of adolescents with depression. *Archives of General Psychiatry, 59*(3), 225–231.

Fergusson, D. M., Horwood, L. J., Ridder, E. M., & Beautrais, A. L. (2005). Subthreshold depression in adolescence and mental health outcomes in adulthood. *Archives of General Psychiatry, 62*(1), 66–72.

Ferster, C. B. (1973). A functional analysis of depression. *American Psychologist, 28*(10), 857–870.

Foa, E. B., & Kozak, M. J. (1986). Emotional processing of fear: Exposure to correct information. *Psychological Bulletin, 99*, 20–35.

Forbes, E. E. (2009). Where's the fun in that?: Broadening the focus on reward function in depression. *Biological Psychiatry, 66*(3), 199–200.

Forbes, E. E., Hariri, A. R., Martin, S. L., Silk, J. S., Moyles, D. L., et al. (2009). Altered striatal activation predicting real-world positive affect in adolescent major depressive disorder. *American Journal of Psychiatry, 166*(1), 64–73.

Garber, J., & Weersing, V. R. (2010). Comorbidity of anxiety and depression in youth: Implications for treatment and prevention. *Clinical Psychology: Science and Practice, 17*, 293–306.

Garland, A. F., Brookman-Frazee, L., Hurlburt, M. S., Accurso, E. C., Zoffness, R. J., Haine-Schlagel, R., et al. (2010). Mental health care for children with disruptive behavior problems: A view inside therapists' offices. *Psychiatric Services, 61*(8), 788–795.

Gaynor, S. T., Lawrence, P. S., & Nelson-Gray, R. O. (2006). Measuring homework compliance in cognitive-behavioral therapy for adolescent depression: Review, preliminary findings, and implications for theory and practice. *Behavior Modification, 30*(5), 647–672.

Gibbons, R., Brown, C., Hur, K., Marcus, S., Bhaumik, D., Erkens, J., et al. (2007). Early evidence on the effects of regulators' suicidality warnings on SSRI prescriptions and suicide in children and adolescents. *American Journal of Psychiatry, 164*(9), 1356–1363.

Giedd, J. N. (2004). Structural magnetic resonance imaging of the adolescent brain. *Annals of the New York Academy of Sciences, 1021*(1), 77–85.

Giedd, J. N., Blumenthal, J., Jeffries, N. O., Castellanos, F. X., Liu, H., Zijdenbos, A., et al. (1999). Brain development during childhood and adolescence: A longitudinal MRI study. *Nature Neuroscience, 2*(10), 861–863.

Glied, S., & Pine, D. S. (2002). Consequences and correlates of adolescent depression. *Archives of Pediatrics and Adolescent Medicine, 156*(10), 1009–1014.

Goodman, J. D., McKay, J. R., & DePhilippis, D. (2013). Progress monitoring in mental health and addiction treatment: A means of improving care. *Professional Psychology: Research and Practice, 44*(4), 231–246.

Goodyer, I. M., Herbert, J., Tamplin, A., & Altham, P. M. E. (2000). First-episode major depression in adolescents affective, cognitive and endocrine characteristics of risk status and predictors of onset. *British Journal of Psychiatry, 176*(2), 142–149.

Gould, E., & Tanapat, P. (1999). Stress and hippocampal neurogenesis. *Biological Psychiatry, 46*(11), 1472–1479.

Gunlicks-Stoessel, M., Mufson, L., Jekal, A., & Turner, J. B. (2010). The impact of perceived interpersonal functioning on treatment for adolescent depression: IPT-A versus treatment as usual in school-based health clinics. *Journal of Consulting and Clinical Psychology, 78*(2), 260–267.

Hankin, B. L., Abramson, L. Y., Moffitt, T. E., Silva, P. A., McGee, R., & Angell, K. E. (1998). Development of depression from preadolescence to young adulthood: Emerging gender differences in a 10-year longitudinal study. *Journal of Abnormal Psychology, 107*(1), 128–140.

Hare, T. A., Tottenham, N., Galván, A., Voss, H. U., Glover, G. H., & Casey, B. J. (2008). Biological substrates of emotional reactivity and regulation in adolescence during an emotional go-nogo task. *Biological Psychiatry, 63*, 927–934.

Helzer, J. E., Kraemer, H. C., & Krueger, R. F. (2006). The feasibility and need for dimensional psychiatric diagnoses. *Psychological Medicine, 36*, 1671–1680.

Henggeler, S. W., Schoenwald, S. K., Borduin, C. M., Rowland, M. D., & Cunningham, P. B. (1998). *Multisystemic treatment of antisocial behavior in children and adolescents*. New York: Guilford Press.

Hlastala, S. A., Kotler, J. S., McClellan, J. M., & McCauley, E. A. (2010). Interpersonal and social rhythm therapy for adolescents with bipolar disorder: Treatment development and results from an open trial. *Depression and Anxiety, 27*(5), 457–464.

Hollon, S. D., Garber, J., & Shelton, R. C. (2005). Treatment of depression in adolescents with cognitive behavior therapy and medications: A commentary on the TADS project. *Cognitive and Behavioral Practice, 12*(2), 149–155.

Israel, P., & Diamond, G. S. (2013). Feasibility of attachment based family therapy for depressed clinic-referred Norwegian adolescents. *Clinical Child Psychology and Psychiatry, 18*(3), 334–350.

Jacob, M. L., Keeley, M., Ritschel, L., & Craighead, W. E. (2013). Behavioural activation for the treatment of low-income, African American adolescents with major depressive disorder: A case series. *Clinical Psychology and Psychotherapy, 20*(1), 87–96.

Jacobson, N. S., Dobson, K. S., Truax, P. A., Addis, M. E., Koerner, K., Gollan, J. K., et al. (1996). A component analysis of cognitive-behavioral treatment for depression. *Journal of Consulting and Clinical Psychology, 64*(2), 295–304.

Jacobson, N. S., Martell, C. R., & Dimidjian, S. (2001). Behavioral activation treatment for depression: Returning to contextual roots. *Clinical Psychology: Science and Practice, 8*(3), 255–270.

Jobes, D. (2006). *Managing suicide risk: A collaborative approach*. New York: Guilford Press.

Kazantzis, N., Deane, F., & Ronan, K. (2000). Homework assignments in cognitive and behavioral therapy: A meta-analysis. *Clinical Psychology: Science and Practice, 7*, 199–202.

Kazantzis, N., Whittington, C., & Dattilio, F. (2010). Meta-analysis of homework effects in cognitive and behavioral therapy: A replication and extension. *Clinical Psychology: Science and Practice, 17*(2), 144–156.

Kazdin, A. E., & Rotella, C. (2013). *The everyday parenting toolkit: The Kazdin method for easy, step-by-step, lasting change for you and your child*. Boston: Houghton Mifflin Harcourt.

Keenan-Miller, D., Hammen, C. L., & Brennan, P. A. (2007). Health outcomes related to early adolescent depression. *Journal of Adolescent Health, 41*(3), 256–262.

Kendall, P., & Beidas, R. (2007). Smoothing the trail for dissemination of evidence-based practices for youth: Flexibility within fidelity. *Professional Psychology: Research and Practice, 38*, 13–20.

Kennard, B. D., Silva, S. G., Tonev, S., Rohde, P., Hughes, J. L., Vitiello, B., et al. (2009). Remission and recovery in the Treatment for Adolescents with Depression Study (TADS): Acute and long-term outcomes. *Journal of the American Academy of Child and Adolescent Psychiatry, 48*(2), 186–195.

Kennard, B. D., Silva, S., Vitiello, B., Curry, J., Kratochvil, C., Simons, A., et al. (2006). Remission and residual symptoms after short-term treatment in the Treatment of Adolescents with Depression Study (TADS). *Journal of the American Academy of Child and Adolescent Psychiatry, 45*(12), 1404–1411.

Kerfoot, M., Harrington, R., Harrington, V., Rogers, J., & Verduyn, C. (2004). A step too far?: Randomized trial of cognitive-behaviour therapy delivered by social workers to depressed adolescents. *European Child and Adolescent Psychiatry, 13*(2), 92–99.

Klein, D. N., Dougherty, L. R., & Olino, T. M. (2005). Toward guidelines for evidence-based assessment of depression in children and adolescents. *Journal of Child and Adolescent Clinical Psychology, 34*, 412–432.

Kraemer, H. C. (2007). DSM categories and dimensions in clinical and research contexts. *International Journal of Methods in Psychiatric Research, 16*(Suppl. 1), S8–S15.

Lambert, M. J., Whipple, J. L., Vermeersch, D. A., Smart, D. W., Hawkins, E. J., Nielsen, S. L., et al. (2002). Enhancing psychotherapy outcomes via providing feedback on client progress: A replication. *Clinical Psychology and Psychotherapy, 9*, 91–103.

Law, M., King, G., King, S., Kertoy, M., Hurley, P., Rosenbaum, P., et al. (2006). Patterns of participation in recreational and leisure activities among children with complex physical disabilities. *Developmental Medicine and Child Neurology, 48*, 337–342.

Lewinsohn, P. M. (1974). Clinical and theoretical aspects of depression. In K. S. Calhoun,

H. E. Adams, & K. M. Mitchell (Eds.), *Innovative treatment methods in psychopathology* (pp. 63–120). New York: Wiley.

Lewinsohn, P. M., Clarke, G. N., Hops, H., & Andrews, J. (1990). Cognitive-behavioral treatment for depressed adolescents. *Behavior Therapy, 21*(4), 385–401.

Lewinsohn, P. M., Clarke, G. N., Seeley, J. R., & Rohde, P. (1994). Major depression in community adolescents: Age at onset, episode duration, and time to recurrence. *Journal of the American Academy of Child and Adolescent Psychiatry, 33*(6), 809–818.

Lewinsohn, P. M., Hops, H., Roberts, R. E., Seeley, J. R., & Andrews, J. A. (1993). Adolescent psychopathology: I. Prevalence and incidence of depression and other DSM-III-R disorders in high school students. *Journal of Abnormal Psychology, 102*(1), 133–144.

Lewinsohn, P. M., Rohde, P., Seeley, J. R., Klein, D. N., & Gotlib, I. H. (2000). Natural course of adolescent major depressive disorder in a community sample: Predictors of recurrence in young adults. *American Journal of Psychiatry, 157*(10), 1584–1591.

Lewinsohn, P. M., Rohde, P., Seeley, J. R., Klein, D. N., & Gotlib, I. H. (2003). Psychosocial functioning of young adults who have experienced and recovered from major depressive disorder during adolescence. *Journal of Abnormal Psychology, 112*(3), 353–363.

Lewinsohn, P. M., Solomon, A., Seeley, J. R., & Zeiss, A. (2000). Clinical implications of "subthreshold" depressive symptoms. *Journal of Abnormal Psychology, 109*(2), 345–351.

Lewis, C. C., Simons, A. D., Nguyen, L. J., Murakami, J. L., Reid, M. W., Silva, S. G., et al. (2010). Impact of childhood trauma on treatment outcome in the Treatment for Adolescents With Depression Study (TADS). *Journal of the American Academy of Child and Adolescent Psychiatry, 49*(2), 132–140.

Libby, A., Brent, D., Morrato, E., Orton, H., Allen, R., & Valuck, R. (2007). Decline in treatment of pediatric depression after FDA advisory on risk of suicidality with SSRIs. *American Journal of Psychiatry, 164*(6), 884–891.

Libby, A. M., Orton, H. D., & Valuck, R. J. (2009). Persisting decline in depression treatment after FDA warnings. *Archives of General Psychiatry, 66*(6), 633–639.

Linehan, M. M. (1993). *Cognitive-behavioral treatment of borderline personality disorder.* New York: Guilford Press.

Linehan, M. M., McCauley, E., Berk, M., & Asarnow, J. (2012, November). *Collaborative adolescent research on emotions and suicide.* Paper presented at the meeting of the Association for Behavioral and Cognitive Theories, National Harbor, MD.

Lo, C. S., Ho, S. M., & Hollon, S. D. (2008). The effects of rumination and negative cognitive styles on depression: A mediation analysis. *Behaviour Research and Therapy, 46*, 487–495.

Lopez, A. D., Mathers, C. D., Ezzati, M., Jamison, D. T., & Murray, C. J. (2006). Global and regional burden of disease and risk factors, 2001: Systematic analysis of population health data. *Lancet, 367*(9524), 1747–1757.

Luna, B., Padmanabhan, A., & O'Hearn, K. (2010). What has fMRI told us about the development of cognitive control through adolescence? *Brain and Cognition, 72*(1), 101–113.

Lyon, A. R., Borntrager, C., Nakamura, B., & Higa-McMillan, C. (2013). From distal to proximal: Routine educational data monitoring in school-based mental health. *Advances in School Mental Health Promotion, 6*(4), 263–279.

Mann, J. J., Emslie, G., Baldessarini, R. J., Beardslee, W., Fawcett, J. A., Goodwin, F. K., et al. (2006). ACNP Task Force report on SSRIs and suicidal behavior in youth. *Neuropsychopharmacology, 31*(3), 473–492.

Martell, C. R., Addis, M. E., & Jacobson, N. S. (2001). *Depression in context: Strategies for guided action.* New York: Norton.

Martin, J., Romas, M., Medford, M., Leffert, N., & Hatcher, S. L. (2006). Adult helping qualities preferred by adolescents. *Adolescence, 41*(161), 127–140.

Maslow, G. R., Haydon, A., McRee, A. L., Ford, C. A., & Halpern, C. T. (2011). Growing up with a chronic illness: Social success, educational/vocational distress. *Journal of Adolescent Health, 49*, 206–212.

McCauley, E., Schloredt, K. A., Gudmundsen, G., Martell, C., Dimidjian, S. (2015). The Adolescent Behavioral Activation Program: Adapting behavioral activation as a treatment for depression in adolescence. *Journal of Clinical Child and Adolescent Psychology*, published online 20/Jan, 2015. *http://dx.doi.org/10.1080/15374416.2014.979933.*

McCauley, E., Schloredt, K., Gudmundsen, G., Martell, C., & Dimidjian, S. (2011). Expanding behavioral activation to depressed adolescents: Lessons learned in treatment development. *Cognitive and Behavioral Practice, 18*, 371–388.

Messer, S. C., Angold, A., Costello, E. J., Loeber, R., Van Kammen, W., & Stouthamer-Loeber, M. (1995). Development of a short questionnaire for use in epidemiological studies of depression in children and adolescents: Factor composition and structure across development. *International Journal of Methods in Psychiatric Research, 5*, 251–262.

Miller, W. R., & Rollnick, S. (2002). *Motivational interviewing: Preparing people for change* (2nd ed.). New York: Guilford Press.

Miller, W. R., Sorensen, J. L., Selzer, J. A., & Brigham, G. S. (2006). Disseminating evidence-based practices in substance abuse treatment: A review with suggestions. *Journal of Substance Abuse Treatment, 31*(1), 25–39.

Moreland, C. S., Bonin, L., Brent, D., & Solomon, D. (2015). Effect of antidepressants on suicide risk in children and adolescents. Wolters Kluwer UpToDate, *www.uptodate.com.*

Mufson, L. (2010). Interpersonal psychotherapy for depressed adolescents (IPT-A): Extending the reach from academic to community settings. *Child and Adolescent Mental Health, 15*(2), 66–72.

Mufson, L., Dorta, K. P., Moreau, D., & Weissman, M. M. (2011). *Interpersonal psychotherapy for depressed adolescents* (2nd ed.). New York: Guilford Press.

Mufson, L., Dorta, K. P., Wickramaratne, P., Nomura, Y., Olfson, M., & Weissman, M. M. (2004). A randomized effectiveness trial of interpersonal psychotherapy for depressed adolescents. *Archives of General Psychiatry, 61*(6), 577–584.

Mufson, L., Weissman, M. M., Moreau, D., & Garfinkel, R. (1999). Efficacy of interpersonal psychotherapy for depressed adolescents. *Archives of General Psychiatry, 56*(6), 573–579.

Naar-King, S., & Suarez, M. (2011). *Motivational interviewing with adolescents and young adults.* New York: Guilford Press.

Nanni, V., Uher, R., & Danese, A. (2012). Childhood maltreatment predicts unfavorable course of illness and treatment outcome in depression: A meta-analysis. *American Journal of Psychiatry, 169*(2), 141–151.

Nemeroff, C. B., Kalali, A., Keller, M. B., Charney, D. S., Lenderts, S. E., Cascade, E. F., et al. (2007). Impact of publicity concerning pediatric suicidality data on physician practice patterns in the United States. *Archives of General Psychiatry, 64*(4), 466–472.

Nock, M., & Ferriter, C. (2005). Parent management of attendance and adherence in child and adolescent therapy: A conceptual and empirical review. *Clinical Child and Family Psychology Review, 8*, 149–166.

Nolen-Hoeksema, S. (2000). The role of rumination in depressive disorder and mixed anxiety/depressive symptoms. *Journal of Abnormal Psychology, 109*, 504–511.

Offidani, E., Fava, G. A., Tomba, E., & Baldessarini, R, J. (2013). Excessive mood elevation and behavioral activation with antidepressant treatment of juvenile depressive and anxiety disorders: A systematic review. *Psychotherapy and Psychosomatics, 82*, 132–141.

Pagoto, S., Bodenlos, J. S., Schneider, K. L., Olendzki, B., & Spates, C. R. (2008). Initial investigation of behavioral activation therapy for co-morbid major depressive disorder and obesity. *Psychotherapy, 45*(3), 410–415.

Palinkas, L., Schoenwald, S., Hoagwood, K., Landsverk, J., Chorpita, B., & Weisz, J. (2008). An ethnographic study of implementation of evidence-based treatments in child mental health: First steps. *Psychiatric Services, 59*(7), 738–746.

Pellerin, K., Costa, N., Weems, C., & Dalton, R. (2010). An examination of treatment completers and non-completers at a child and adolescent community mental health clinic. *Community Mental Health Journal, 46*(3), 273–281.

Persons, J. B. (2008). *The case formulation approach to cognitive-behavior therapy.* New York: Guilford Press.

Piacentini, J., March, J., & Franklin, M. (2006). Cognitive-behavioral therapy for youngsters with obsessive–compulsive disorder. In P. C. Kendall (Ed.), *Child and adolescent therapy: Cognitive-behavioral procedures* (3rd ed., pp. 297–321). New York: Guilford Press.

Reynolds, W. M. (1987). *Suicide Ideation Questionnaire: Professional manual.* Odessa, FL: Psychological Assessment Resources.

Richardson, L. P., DiGiuseppe, D., Christakis, D. A., McCauley, E., & Katon, W. (2004). Quality of care for Medicaid-covered youth treated with antidepressant therapy. *Archives of General Psychiatry, 61*(5), 475–480.

Richardson, L. P., & Katzenellenbogen, R. (2005). Childhood and adolescent depression: The role of primary care providers in diagnosis and treatment. *Current Problems in Pediatric and Adolescent Health Care, 35,* 6–24.

Richardson, L. P., McCauley, E., Grossman, D. C., McCarty, C. A., Richards, J., Russo, J. E., et al. (2010). Evaluation of the Patient Health Questionnaire–9 Item for detecting major depression among adolescents. *Pediatrics, 126*(6), 1117–1123.

Ritschel, L. A., Ramirez, C. L., Jones, M., & Craighead, W. E. (2011). Behavioral activation for depressed teens: A pilot study. *Cognitive and Behavioral Practice, 18*(2), 281–299.

Rosselló, J., & Bernal, G. (1999). The efficacy of cognitive-behavioral and interpersonal treatments for depression in Puerto Rican adolescents. *Journal of Consulting and Clinical Psychology, 67*(5), 734–745.

Rotheram-Borus, M. J., Swendeman, D., & Chorpita, B. F. (2012). Disruptive innovations for designing and diffusing evidence-based interventions. *American Psychologist, 67*(6), 463–476.

Ryba, M. M., Lejuez, C. W., & Hopko, D. R. (2014). Behavioral activation for depressed breast cancer patients: The impact of therapeutic compliance and quantity of activities completed on symptom reduction. *Journal of Consulting and Clinical Psychology, 82*(2), 325–335.

Shirk, S. R., & Karver, M. (2003). Prediction of treatment outcome from relationship variables in child and adolescent therapy: A meta-analytic review. *Journal of Consulting and Clinical Psychology, 71*(3), 452–464.

Siegle, G. J., Steinhauer, S. R., Friedman, E. S., Thompson, W. S., & Thase, M. E. (2011). Remission prognosis for cognitive therapy for recurrent depression using the pupil: Utility and neural correlates. *Biological Psychiatry, 69*(8), 726–733.

Silk, J. S., Dahl, R. E., Ryan, N. D., Forbes, E. E., Axelson, D. A., Birmaher, B., et al. (2007). Pupillary reactivity to emotional information in child and adolescent depression: Links to clinical and ecological measures. *American Journal of Psychiatry, 164*(12), 1873–1880.

Simon, G. E. (2006). The antidepressant quandary—considering suicide risk when treating adolescent depression. *New England Journal of Medicine, 355*(26), 2722–2723.

Skinner, B. F. (1953). *Science and human behavior.* New York: Free Press.

Slavich, G. M. (2014, October 11). *Depression from a social neuroimmunologic perspective.* Paper presented at the meeting Neuroscience of Youth Depression, University of North Carolina, Chapel Hill, NC.

Somerville, L. H., Jones, R. M., & Casey, B. J. (2010). A time of change: Behavioral and neural correlates of adolescent sensitivity to appetitive and aversive environmental cues. *Brain and Cognition, 72*(1), 124–133.

Soni, A. (2009). *Statistical Brief #248: The five most costly conditions, 1996 and 2006: Estimates for the U.S. civilian noninstitutionalized population*. Rockville, MD: Agency for Healthcare Research and Quality.

Stam, H., Hartman, E. E., Deurloo, J. A., Groothoff, J., & Grootenhuis, M. A. (2006). Young adult patients with a history of pediatric disease: Impact on course of life and transition into adulthood. *Journal of Adolescent Health, 39*, 4–13.

Steinberg, L., Dahl, R., Keating, D., Kupfer, D. J., Masten, A. S., & Pine, D. S. (2006). The study of developmental psychopathology in adolescence: Integrating affective neuroscience with the study of context. In D. Cicchetti & D. Cohen (Eds.), *Developmental psychopathology: Vol. 2. Developmental neuroscience* (pp. 710–741). New York: Wiley.

TADS (Treatment for Adolescents with Depression Study) Team. (2003). Treatment for Adolescents with Depression Study (TADS): Rationale, design, and methods. *Journal of the American Academy of Child and Adolescent Psychiatry, 42*(5), 531–542.

TADS (Treatment for Adolescents with Depression Study) Team. (2004). Fluoxetine, cognitive-behavioral therapy, and their combination for adolescents with depression: Treatment for adolescents with depression study (TADS) randomized controlled trial. *Journal of the American Medical Association, 292*(7), 807–820.

TADS (Treatment for Adolescents with Depression Study) Team. (2007). The Treatment for Adolescents with Depression Study (TADS): Long-term effectiveness and safety outcomes. *Archives of General Psychiatry, 64*(10), 1132–1144.

Thapar, A., Collishaw, S., Pine, D. S., & Thapar, A. K. (2012). Depression in adolescence. *Lancet, 379*(9820), 1056–1067.

Treynor, W., Gonzalez, R., & Nolen-Hoeksema, S. (2003). Rumination reconsidered: A psychometric analysis. *Cognitive Therapy and Research, 27*, 247–259.

Velanova, K., Wheeler, M. E., & Luna, B. (2008). Maturational changes in anterior cingulate and frontoparietal recruitment support the development of error processing and inhibitory control. *Cerebral Cortex, 18*(11), 2505–2522.

Weisz, J. R., Chorpita, B. F., Palinkas, L. A., Schoenwald, S. K., Miranda, J., Bearman, S. K., et al. (2012). Testing standard and modular designs for psychotherapy treating depression, anxiety, and conduct problems in youth: A randomized effectiveness trial. *Archives of General Psychiatry, 69*(3), 274–282.

Weisz, J. R., Jensen, A. L., & McLeod, B. D. (2005). Development and dissemination of child and adolescent psychotherapies: Milestones, methods, and a new deployment-focused model. In E. D. Hibbs & P. S. Jensen (Eds.), *Psychosocial treatment for child and adolescent disorders: Empirically based strategies for clinical practice* (2nd ed.) (pp. 9–39). Washington, DC: American Psychological Association.

Weisz, J. R., Jensen-Doss, A., & Hawley, K. M. (2006). Evidence-based youth psychotherapies versus usual clinical care: A meta-analysis of direct comparisons. *American Psychologist, 61*, 671–689.

Weisz, J. R., Kuppens, S., Eckshtain, D., Ugueto, A. M., Hawley, K. M., & Jensen-Doss, A. (2013). Performance of evidence-based youth psychotherapies compared with usual clinical care: A multilevel meta-analysis. *JAMA Psychiatry, 70*(7), 750–761.

Williams, R. A., Hollis, H. M., & Benoit, K. (1998). Attitudes toward psychiatric medications among incarcerated female adolescents. *Journal of the American Academy of Child and Adolescent Psychiatry, 37*(12), 1301–1307.

Wolff, J. C., & Ollendick, T. H. (2006). The comorbidity of conduct problems and depression in childhood and adolescence. *Clinical Child and Family Psychology Review, 9*, 201–220.

Young, J. F., Mufson, L., & Davies, M. (2006). Efficacy of Interpersonal Psychotherapy–Adolescent Skills Training: An indicated preventive intervention for depression. *Journal of Child Psychology and Psychiatry, 47*(12), 1254–1262.

Index

Note. A page number in italics indicates a figure or a table.

A-BAP modules
   "Getting Active," 47–50, 105–120
   "Getting Started," 44–47, 89–104
   "Moving Forward," 56, 165–171
   overview, 11, *12–13*, 43–44
   "Practice," 55–56, 153–163
   "Skill Building," 50–55, 121–151
   See also individual modules
A-BAP sessions
   "Goal-Directed Behavior versus Mood-Directed Behavior," 47–48, 107–113
   "Goal Setting," 51–53, 131–137
   "Identifying Barriers," 53, 138–144
   "Introducing Consequences of Behavior," 48–50, 114–120
   "Introduction to A-BAP," 44–46, 91–96
   "Overcoming Avoidance," 54–55, 145–151
   overview, 10–14, 43–44
   "Practicing Skills," 55–56, 160–163
   "Putting It All Together," 55–56, 155–159
   "Relapse Prevention and Saying Good-Bye," 56, 167–171
   "Situation–Activity–Mood Cycle," 46–47, 97–104
   structure of, 14, *15*
   See also individual sessions
"Action Plan" handout, 56, 156, 161, 162–163, 168, 169, 170, 171, 210
Active listening, 51, 128–129
"Activities Menu" teaching guide, 49, 115, 118, 189
"Activities That Help to PUMP You Up!" handout, 50, 115, 119–120, 124, 125, 190
Activity
   activity–mood monitoring, 111–112
   impact on mood, 99–100
   monitoring, 95–96
   "pump you up" versus "bring you down," 49, 50, 66, 80, 118
   situation–activity–mood cycle, 46–47, 100–101

"Activity Monitoring" handout, 46, 92, 96, 98, 99, 177
"Activity–Mood Chart—Example" worksheet, 48, 108, 109, 111, 184
"Activity–Mood Chart" worksheet, 48, 108, 109, 111–112, 115, 116, 185
Adolescent Behavioral Activation Program (A-BAP)
   case conceptualization, 30–40
   collaborating with the adolescent and enhancing motivation for change, 21–22
   considerations regarding appropriate candidates for, 24–25
   efficacy of, 9–10
   extending to other populations
      overview and summary, 75, 85
      young or cognitively immature individuals, 84–85
      youth with medical problems, 81–84
      youth with other psychopathology, 75–81
   integration with other therapeutic strategies, 57–58
   key intervention strategies
      functional analysis, 17–18
      overcoming avoidance, 18
      overview, 15–16
      reinforcement, 16–17
      structural elements, 18–20
   multitrait, multimethod (MTMM) assessment, 26–30
   overview, 1–2, 10–15, 23
   parental involvement, 20–21 (*see also* Parents)
   rationale for, 8–9
   treatment challenges
      engagement issues, 59–67
      escalation of distress and symptoms, 67–72
      family and/or environmental circumstances, 72–74
      summary, 74
   treatment planning, 40–42
Adolescent depression
   current approaches to treating, 3–6
   problem of, 2–3
Adult depression, behavioral activation for, 8

Anger, 79
  See also "Bursting"
Anxiety, 76–79
Assessment. *See* Multitrait, multimethod (MTMM) assessment
Attachment-based family therapy (ABFT), 4
Attendance issues, 60–62
Attention-deficit/hyperactivity disorder (ADHD), 76
Avoidance
  concept and discussion of, 18
  emphasis on in behavioral activation, 7
  overcoming, 18, 54–55, 148–150
  recognizing that avoidance works, 148
  understanding, 147–148

Barriers, recognizing and getting around, 53, 140–142
"Barriers: Internal versus External" teaching guide, 53, 58, 139, 141, 202
Behavior
  goal-directed versus mood-directed, 47–48
  payoff versus price concept, 49, 116–117
  rehearsal/practice in A-BAP, 19
Behavioral activation (BA)
  for adolescent depression, 8–9
  for adult depression, 8
  behavioral model of depression, 7
  integration with other therapeutic strategies, 57–58
  key intervention strategies, 15–20
  See also Adolescent Behavioral Activation Program
"Behavioral Activation Model" teaching guide, 45, 92, 94, 175
Biased cognitive processing, 6
Brooding, 65
"Bursting," 54, 69, 79, 147–148

Case conceptualization
  overview, 30–31
  treatment planning and, 40
  vignettes illustrating, 31–40
CBT. *See* Cognitive-behavioral therapy
Child Behavior Checklist (CBCL), 29
Chronic illness, 81–82
Coaching stance, of the therapist in A-BAP, 10, 21–22, 45, 60
Cognitive-behavioral therapy (CBT)
  for adolescent depression, 3–4, 5–6
  behavioral activation and, 7
  difficulties in disseminating, 8–9
  homework adherence and, 19
  integration of A-BAP with, 57–58
Cognitive immaturity, A-BAP and, 84–85
Cognitive restructuring, 6
Cognitive therapy (CT), 8
Collaboration, in A-BAP, 21–22
"Communicating with Support: What Can You Do to Help an Interaction Go Well" handout, 51, 124, 129, 195
Communication, parents and active listening, 51, 128–129
Consequences of behavior
  introducing, 48–50
  short-term versus long-term, 49, 117
Contextual factors, collecting information about, 29–30
COPE (Calm and Clarify, Options, Perform, Evaluate)
  in anxiety interventions, 78
  with cognitively immature youth, 85
  with highly reactive youth, 43–44
  in interventions for disruptive behavior, 79
  in managing "crisis of the week" scenarios, 69
  in "Overcoming Avoidance" session, 54
  in "Problem Solving" session, 51
  reviewing, 133
  using to handle challenging situations and manage stress, 125–128
"Crisis of the week" scenarios, challenges with managing, 67–69

Depression
  in adults, behavioral activation for, 8
  behavioral activation model of, 7
  See also Adolescent depression
Depression Timeline, 29–30, *30*
"Developing an Action Plan" handout, 56, 156, 209
Dialectic behavior therapy (DBT), 70, 71
Disruptive behavior, 79–81
Doing What Works, 170
"Doing What Works" worksheet, 56, 168, 170, 171, 211
"Downward Spiral, Upward Spiral" handout, 47, 98, 100–101, 179

Engagement issues
  attendance, 60–62
  homework completion, 63–64
  initial engagement and rapport building, 60
  motivation to change, 64–66
  overview and summary of, 59–60, 66–67
  treatment targets, 66
Environmental circumstances, challenges with managing, 72–74
Escalation of distress, challenges of, 67–72
Exposure-based interventions, 77

Family circumstances, challenges with managing, 72–74
Family conflict, challenges of managing, 74
Functional analysis, 17–28

"Gateway" disorders, 27
Generalized anxiety disorder (GAD), 76
"Getting Active" module
  concepts and skills introduced in, 47–50
  description of sessions, 105–120
  overview, 11, *12*
"Getting Active!" teaching guide, 47, 108, 109, 110, 139, 140, 141–142, 183
"Getting Started" module
  concepts and skills introduced in, 44–47
  description of sessions, 91–104
  overview, 11, *12*
Goal-directed behavior, versus mood-directed behavior, 47–48
"Goal-Directed Behavior versus Mood-Directed Behavior" session
  agenda, 108–109
  concepts and skills introduced in, 47–48
  outline, 109–113
  overview, *12*, 107–108
Goals
  recognizing and getting around barriers to, 53, 140–142
  "SMART" goals, 51–52, 55, 78, 134–135
"Goals and Barriers" handout, 53, 139, 140, 142, 146, 147, 156, 203

Index

Goal setting
   in A-BAP, 51–53, 134–135
   setting a new goal and identifying mini-steps to achieving, 52, 142
"Goal Setting" session
   agenda, 132–133
   concepts and skills introduced in, 51–53
   outline, 133–137
   overview, *12*, 131–132
"Goal Setting" worksheet, 52, 53, 78, 132, 133, 135, 139, 140, 199
Good feelings, making the most of, 119–120

Handouts
   purpose of, 44
   See also individual handouts, worksheets, or teaching guides
"Hibernating," 54, 148
High-risk behaviors, challenges with managing, 70
Homework
   CBT and, 19
   completion issues, 63–64
   See also "Test It Out" activities
"How Behavioral Activation Works for You" worksheet, 45, 55, 92, 94–95, 156, 157, 158, 176
"How SMART Is This Goal?" teaching guide, 51–52, 132, 134, 197
"How to Communicate with Support" teaching guide, 51, 124, 129, 193

"Identifying a SMART Goal" worksheet, 51–52, 132, 134–135, 198
"Identifying Barriers" session
   agenda, 139–140
   concepts and skills introduced in, 53
   outline, 140–144
   overview, *13*, 138–139
Interpersonal therapy (IPT)
   integration of A-BAP with, 57–58
   treatment of adolescent depression, 3, 4, 5–6
"Introducing Consequences of Behavior" session
   agenda, 115
   concepts and skills introduced in, 48–50
   outline, 116–120
   overview, *12*, 114–115
"Introduction to A-BAP" session
   agenda, 92
   concepts and skills introduced in, 44–46
   outline, 93–96
   overview, *12*, 91–92

Modularized approaches to treating adolescent depression, 6
Monitoring
   of activity, 95–96
   activity–mood monitoring, 111–112
   and strategies for providing ongoing support by parents, 136–137, 143, 150–151
   of symptoms in A-BAP, 18–19
"Monitoring Support" handout, 53, 132, 133, 137, 139, 143, 201
Mood
   activity–mood monitoring, 111–112
   bolstering, 49–50
   how relationships and activities impact, 46–47, 99–100
   situation–activity–mood cycle, 46–47, 100–101
   using activity to improve, 109–110
Mood-directed behavior, versus goal-directed behavior, 47–48
Motivational Interviewing (MI), 22, 64, 70
Motivation to change
   challenges with, 64–66
   enhancing in A-BAP, 22
"Moving Forward" module
   concepts and skills introduced in, 56
   description of sessions, 165–171
   overview, 11, *13*
Multitrait, multimethod (MTMM) assessment
   developmental status of the adolescent, 28–29
   gathering data from various informants, 27–28
   rationale for using with A-BAP, 26
   scope of differential diagnosis and co-occurring disorders, 26–27
   tools for symptom assessment, 29–30

Negative punishment, 16
Negative reinforcement, 16
Nonsupportive parents, challenges with managing, 72–74

Oppositional defiant disorder (ODD), 76
"Overcoming Avoidance" session
   agenda, 146
   concepts and skills introduced in, 54–55
   outline, 147–151
   overview, *13*, 145–146

"A Parent Guide to Adolescent Depression" worksheet, 47, 98, 101–103, 109, 180–182
Parents
   challenges with agreement concerning treatment targets and, 66
   family conflict issues and, 74
   involvement in A-BAP, 20–21
      communication and active listening, 51, 128–129
      monitoring and strategies for providing ongoing support, 136–137, 143, 150–151
      relapse prevention plan, action plan, and saying good-bye, 171
      supporting the adolescent through depression, 103, 112–113
      understanding depression in adolescence, 101–103
   involvement in treatments for adolescent depression, 4
   nonsupportive of activation approaches, challenges with managing, 72–74
   "Test It Out" activities
      "Communicating with Support: What Can You Do to Help an Interaction Go Well," 51, 129–130
      "Monitoring Support," 137
      "Support Experiment," 53, 143, 150–151
      "Ways to Support My Adolescent," 52–53, 136–137
Patient Health Questionnaire-9 (PHQ-9), 14, 29, 70
Payoff versus price concept, 49, 116–117
Pharmacotherapy, 4–5
Positive punishment, 16
Positive reinforcement, 16
"Practice" module
   concepts and skills introduced in, 55–56
   description of sessions, 153–163
   overview, 11, *13*
Practice Wise Managing and Adapting Practice (MAP) system, 6

"Practicing How to Communicate with Support"
worksheet, 51, 124, 129, 194
"Practicing Skills" session
agenda, 161
concepts and skills introduced in, 55–56
outline, 161–163
overview, *13*, 160–161
Problem solving, 51
reflective, 65
See also COPE
"Problem Solving" session
agenda, 124
concepts and skills introduced in, 51
outline, 125–130
overview, *12*, 123–124
"Pump You Up, Bring You Down" worksheet, 49, 58, 115, 118, 188
Punishment, 16
"Putting It All Together" session
agenda, 156
concepts and skills introduced in, 55–56
outline, 157–159
overview, *13*, 155–156

Rapport building issues, 60
Reflective problem solving, 65
Reinforcement, 16–17
Relapse
prevention, 11, 56, 167–168
problem of, 2
"Relapse Prevention and Saying Good-Bye" session
agenda, 168–169
concepts and skills introduced in, 56
outline, 169–171
overview, *13*, 167–168
Relationships
challenges to forming the therapeutic alliance, 60
developmental challenges in adolescence, 28–29
impact on mood, 46–47, 99–100
Response-contingent positive reinforcement (RCPR), 16–17, 40, 41, 42
Review, 162
Rumination, 54, 65–66

Self-harming behaviors, challenges with managing, 70
"Setting SMART Goals" teaching guide, 51, 132, 134, 196
Short Moods and Feelings Questionnaire (SMFQ), 29
"Short- versus Long-Term Consequences" teaching guide, 49, 115, 117, 187
Situation–activity–mood cycle, 46–47, 100–101
"Situation–Activity–Mood Cycle" session
agenda, 98
concepts and skills introduced in, 46–47
outline, 99–104
overview, *12*, 97–98
Skill building, in A-BAP, 19–20
"Skill Building" module
concepts and skills introduced in, 50–55
description of sessions, 121–151
overview, 11, *12–13*
Sleep habits, 28
Slips, 56, 168, 169
"SMART" goals, 51–52, 55, 78, 134–135
Social phobia, 76

Suicidality
challenges with managing, 70–72
treatment with A-BAP, 25
Suicide Ideation Questionnaire (SIQ), 29, 70
"Support Experiment" handout, 53, 55, 139, 140, 143, 146, 150–151, 205
"Support Ideas" teaching guide, 53, 139, 140, 143, 204
Symptoms
challenges of escalation, 67–72
monitoring in A-BAP, 18–19

Taking stock, 157
"Taking Stock" worksheet, 55, 156, 157–158, 208
Termination
in A-BAP, 56, 167–171
note on timing, 57
"Test It Out" activities
"Action Plan," 56, 158, 162–163, 170
"Activities That Help to PUMP You Up!", 50, 119–120
"Activity Monitoring," 46, 96, 99
"Activity–Mood Chart," 48, 111–112
"Developing an Action Plan," 56
"Downward Spiral, Upward Spiral," 47, 101, 109
in the final session, 56
"Goal and Barriers," 53, 142
"Goal Setting," 52, 135
introducing to the adolescent, 46
overview, 14
purpose of, 45
trying out new behaviors and, 19
"Using COPE," 51, 128
"Using TRAP-TRAC to Conquer Avoidance and Overcome the Downward Spiral," 54–55, 150
Therapeutic alliance, challenges to forming, 60
Therapists, coaching stance in A-BAP, 10, 21–22, 45, 60
TRAP-TRAC (Trigger, Response, Avoidance Pattern–Trigger, Response, Alternative Coping), 54–55, 70, 82, 148–150
Treatment of Adolescents with Depression Study (TADS), 3, 9
Treatment planning, overview and discussion of, 40–42
Treatment targets, challenges with agreement concerning, 66

"Using COPE" handout, 51, 124, 128, 132, 133, 192
"Using COPE to Solve Problems" teaching guide, 51, 124, 126–128, 191
"Using TRAP-TRAC to Conquer Avoidance and Overcome the Downward Spiral" worksheet, 54, 58, 146, 149–150, 156, 157, 158, 207

"Ways to Describe Parenting and Adolescent" worksheet, 48, 108, 109, 112–113, 186
"Ways to Support My Adolescent" worksheet, 52–53, 132, 133, 136, 200
Weight management, 82–84
"What Does Avoidance Look Like?" teaching guide, 54, 146, 147–148, 206
"Who and What Is on 'First' in Your Life?" worksheet, 46, 98, 99–100, 178

Youth
with medical problems, A-BAP and, 81–84
with other psychopathology, A-BAP and, 75–81
Youth Self-Report Form (YSR), 29